Who Wants Normal?

'Fierce, funny and so important to disabled women of all ages. A beautiful book of solidarity and feminism when you need it most. I bloody loved it' Ruth Madeley

'Disability is an unnecessarily awkward subject for far too many people given the millions and millions of people within our society who engage with it daily, either due to their own health struggles or those of someone they love. Frances has a talent for destigmatizing the conversation and pushing past the uncomfortable to the necessary in an engaging and undeniable fashion. An inimitable voice in disability advocacy. We all need this book' Jameela Jamil

'Illuminating and spirited – such a necessary book' Marina Hyde

'Frances has long been one of my writing heroes – this book is typically smart, funny, clarifying and enraging' Eva Wiseman

'One of the most interesting and important writers working in the UK today' Nish Kumar

'A razor-sharp, super-smart manifesto by one of the most essential voices in Britain today. This guide is a crucial call to action not just for disabled women, but for everyone who wants to have a better understanding of what it means to live with a disability' Yomi Adegoke

'This superb book is a rallying cry for true equality for disabled people. Full of shocking stats, real life experiences and humour, it made me angry, laugh and gasp' Victoria Derbyshire

'I've never related to a book more. Brilliant, honest and so powerful. Disabled or not, you MUST read this book' Rosie Jones

'The must-read manifesto . . . this new book blends memoir and practical insight in an unmissable call to action . . . it covers education, careers, health, body image, relationships, representation and more' *Stylist*, '26 must-read books that will be massive this year'

'There are so many "Yes! That happened to me too!" moments in this book that reading it feels like having a gossipy evening in with the best of friends – the best disabled women friends' Liz Carr

'This book is beautiful, vital and important. I loved it' Jack Thorne

By the same author

Crippled: Austerity and the Demonization
of Disabled People

Who Wants Normal?

The Disabled Girls' Guide to Life

FRANCES RYAN

FIG TREE
an imprint of
PENGUIN BOOKS

FIG TREE

UK | USA | Canada | Ireland | Australia
India | New Zealand | South Africa

Fig Tree is part of the Penguin Random House group of companies
whose addresses can be found at global.penguinrandomhouse.com.

Penguin Random House UK,
One Embassy Gardens, 8 Viaduct Gardens, London SW11 7BW

penguin.co.uk

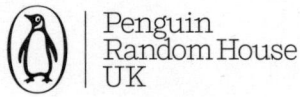

Penguin
Random House
UK

First published 2025
001

Set in 11.6/15.8pt Calluna
Typeset by Jouve (UK), Milton Keynes
Printed and bound in Great Britain by Clays Ltd, Elcograf S.p.A.

The authorized representative in the EEA is Penguin Random House Ireland,
Morrison Chambers, 32 Nassau Street, Dublin D02 YH68

A CIP catalogue record for this book is available from the British Library

ISBN: 978-0-241-62943-7

Penguin Random House is committed to a sustainable future
for our business, our readers and our planet. This book is made from
Forest Stewardship Council® certified paper.

For Bea – may you never settle for normal

Contents

Contents

WITH THANKS TO

Dr Hannah Barham-Brown

Emma Barnett

Genevieve Barr

Dame Anne Begg

Andrea Begley

Trishna Bharadia

Kit Bithell

Luce Brett

Suzanne Bull MBE

Sinéad Burke

Dr Angharad Butler-Rees

Baroness Jane Campbell

Victoria Canal

Rachel Charlton-Dailey

Dr Stella Chatzitheochari

Dr Sarah Chave

Dr Katharine Cheston

Fearne Cotton

Emilie Cousins

Sarah Deason

Rt Hon. Marsha de Cordova MP

Natasha Devon MBE

Shani Dhanda

Dr Helen Dring-Turner

Prof. Bethan Evans

Rosie Fletcher

Nikki Fox

Ione Gamble

Josie George

Ruth Golding

Ellie Goldstein

Mollie Goodfellow

Sarah Gordy MBE

Baroness Tanni Grey-Thompson

Dr Deepti Gurdasani

Jane Hatton

Anna HeardinLondon

Ali Hirsz

Cherylee Houston MBE

Nikki Jack

Jameela Jamil

Rosie Jones

Dr Amy Kavanagh

Kelly Knox

Dr Kirsty Liddiard

Natasha Lipman

Zoe Lloyd

Ruth Madeley

Marina, formerly Marina and the Diamonds

Amelia McLoughlan

Jillian Mercado

Rachael Mole

Sophie Morgan

Baroness Emma Nicholson

Joanna Owen

Lara Parker

Hannah Jane Parkinson

Fleur Perry

Katie Piper OBE

Stefanie Reid MBE

Samantha Renke

Jenny Sealey OBE

Dr Emma Sheppard

Pippa Stacey

Evie Torrance

Lucy Watts MBE

Rosie Weatherley

Lucy Webster

Lib Whitfield

Nadia Whittome MP

Dr Sula Windgassen

Laura Winson

Alice Wong

Introduction

I am sitting with a ventilator strapped to my face. The air pushes into my chest, the muscles contracting and stretching. In and out. In and out. I am afraid to take it off; that my lungs alone can no longer handle the most basic human functioning. I am afraid to leave it on; that the air will somehow stop flowing from the machine, or worse, that I will never be able to take it off. That I will live like this forever. Or as long as forever feels. Gasping for air, I consider taking up smoking. For the stress.

I would like to be able to start this story with a stellar anecdote about how exactly my life imploded. 'I was walking down Sunset Boulevard and Harry Styles ran me down in a Ferrari.' 'I was dancing on a podium in Ibiza when a falling speaker semi-decapitated me.' In reality, it was much more mundane, as these things inevitably tend to be. I went to the pub and I caught the flu. That was it. Oh sorry – I also got an entire bottle of wine for £12. I remember that detail clearly. I went to the pub, I got drunk on cheap wine, and I caught the flu.

I spent Christmas '17 with what I thought was a regular illness. By February, I was unable to breathe or move. The flu had become flu complications and I had become strapped to a ventilator mask. My energy all but disappeared to the extent that even breathing was a high-end task. In my bedroom, alone, plastic casing enveloped my skin. I looked like Darth Vader, if Darth Vader spent a lot of time in Primark pyjamas. The cliché during this sort of thing is to say that the months that followed were a blur. But as anyone who has ever been through anything knows, really, it is the opposite. You *wish* it were a blur. You would pay good money for a haze, to black out for as long as it takes to get through the worst and to re-emerge fabulous, like a contestant in a Netflix makeover show.

The days did not blur. Each minute was sharpened, as if I was living in a new reality that had been cut out with lasers. I couldn't leave my house, I could barely get out of bed, and I didn't understand any part of that.

Fatigue is hard to comprehend until you have it. I learned abruptly that it was not being tired from a big night out or burnout after a stressful spell at work. It was all-consuming, as if my body were wearing a weighted blanket that I couldn't shake off. Getting up from a toilet was enough to make my knees buckle, pills and dignity draining down the bottom of the sink. For a while, I was surviving off cookies; my narrowed oesophagus refusing to swallow anything else, every muscle now apparently a toddler knee-deep in a tantrum.

Born with a muscle weakness, I was familiar with my body falling short of society's standards. I had used a wheelchair since I was old enough to reach the wheels and had grown up happy and accomplished. I always thought that meant I had a pretty good handle on my health but it turns out I was merely a novice. If my body was a white good, at this point I would have been asking to speak to the manager.

As the months went on, I waited for 'recovery' – that thing that is meant to follow falling ill. I looked out the window each day, twitching the curtain when recovery began to run late. It never came. Instead, the fatigue and pain hung around, like a noxious smell. There was some improvement – my legs no longer buckled when asked to stand – and yet not enough. In bed, I looked through photographs on my camera-roll for evidence of my former life. I traced the timeline on repeat in an attempt to make sense of it. Just a few months earlier I had been out at midnight singing at a gig with an old friend. Now, I had a 'pill basket' and knew the weights of gateway opioids. I was running a daily marathon just to exist, except I could barely recognize the existence. In the four walls of my bedroom, my days had shrunk to fit inside. Seasons passed, the sun crept through the blinds, and I blinked into tomorrow. I'd barely hit thirty and it felt like my life had ended. In my sheets, I held myself. It seemed the polite thing to do.

When your entire world feels like it has fallen in on itself, you tend to cling to any hint of normality. For me, it was my job. Working as a journalist became something to focus on, a lost part of myself I could still find in the dark. I don't want to call it delusion but there was probably a fair hint of that. Besides, I needed to feel something other than sickness. I needed to believe there was going to be more to the rest of my life than simply being ill. I made myself a plan. I would try writing for ten minutes in a morning. Then twenty. If I got dizzy, I would stop.

Two years after falling ill, I had an award-winning column in a national newspaper, my first book was published to critical acclaim, and I was being named one of Britain's most influential disabled people. It had also been so long since I had washed my hair that my scalp was forming its own paste. Perhaps I was a fraud. Perhaps I was in denial. Or perhaps – go with me here – life is much more complicated than they tell you. Perhaps boxes like 'normal' and 'success' are tricks to trap us and a day can be meaningful, hard and funny all at once. Perhaps it is possible to have a body that is unruly, broken, bruised and to actually be OK. To be bloody spectacular. To pick the shards of the broken vase off the floor and super-glue life back together, marvelling at the scent of the flowers (and then find a plaster for the blood).

No one really talks about it. No one really talks about what it is to be a disabled woman, especially a young one. To go through something transformative before you can legally drink. To experience pain or exhaustion or to feel

xvi

ninety-two. To navigate all the standard parts of life – exams, careers, relationships – but with a body that is different from everyone else's. If we do ever share this, we are expected to sanitize it; to dress up disability and sickness in a palatable bow. Even as I write this I am reticent to share the details of my own experience, not simply because it is private but because it runs against how disabled women are told to speak. We learn early on which parts of ourselves can be shared with the world and which parts we must hide, lest we be pitied, rejected or shamed. We are allowed to talk about our disabled bodies only if and when we have managed to make them appear like 'normal' ones. Everyone wants to share the TikTok of the girl rising from her wheelchair to dance at the school prom, not when she feels the music pinprick her skin as she sits. I think it's time that changed.

When I grew up as a disabled teenager in the late 1990s, I knew no other disabled women like me. I'd seen barely a handful on TV and next to none in films. Women's mags portrayed perfection, and sickness and disability seemingly had no part in that. Being a disabled girl wasn't 'normal', was the message, and it was best kept behind closed doors. In some ways, it doesn't feel much better now. Research shows disabled people account for barely 1 per cent of the House of Commons,[1] while the same percentage of those working in the UK media have a disability. It's estimated disabled people make up only 2.5 per cent of people on our television screens,[2] while just 3.4 per cent of children's books have a disabled main character.[3]

Even so-called diversity campaigns often ignore disabled women. In recent years, the much applauded Fenty Beauty launch, marketed with a self-declared commitment to 'exclude no one',[4] championed models of every beautiful colour, size, and faith – but no disability. Apparently, 'exclusion' is OK if it is disabled women. Similarly, British *Vogue*'s celebrated spread in 2018 to mark 100 years since women gained the vote gloriously gave a platform to black, Muslim, and trans women – but not a disabled one.[5] There has been some improvement in the last few years – for its part, *Vogue* did a disability special in 2023 – but it is still all too rare to see women with disabilities on the beauty pages. Meanwhile, brands and companies that rightly put out marketing for (LGBTQ+) Pride or International Women's Day are strangely silent when Disability Pride month comes around. (That disabled people are also gay, people of colour, trans or young is also routinely ignored.)

In the few times disability is featured in popular culture, it is still largely simplistic or outright bleak. Read a newspaper and you'll see a disabled person described as 'suffering' from their condition. Click on Instagram and someone will be having a good cry because they watched a woman using a cane 'bravely' leave the house. On the other hand, if you see disabled people 'succeeding', they are generally presented as doing well 'despite' their disability. They are superhuman – their disability or illness is something they have 'overcome', an abstract concept unencumbered by unappealing reality like pills and pain. 'I don't see your disability' is a common well-meaning phrase by non-disabled people, as if it were a compliment to suggest a key part of ourselves should be erased. As disabled people, our choice is binary: to be open about our health and be labelled 'inspirational' – or worse, faking – or to hide it from view entirely. Disabled women, for our part, are simultaneously defined by sexism and ableism. We are waif or warrior, infantilized or invisible. Meanwhile, disabled people are represented as a set demographic: typically white, usually male, often old and retired or a wheelchair user. Women with disabilities – let alone disabled women of colour, trans, or young – are often left out of popular culture entirely.

The exclusion of disabled women is not simply representational – disabled women are, quite literally, physically shut out of everyday life. Despite the UK having anti-discrimination laws that give rights to disabled people, society is still too often designed for non-disabled bodies. Nearly a third of disabled people say they find using public spaces difficult 'all the time' or 'often', according to the UK Disability Survey in 2021.[6] Outdated transport takes away our freedom to move around and travel; a survey in 2022 found none of the ten busiest train stations in the UK are fully accessible,[7] while only a third of the Tube stations on the London Underground are suitable for wheelchair users.[8] If you're physically disabled, even your – or other people's – homes are often impossible to get in or live in safely; only 9 per cent of English housing provides the most basic accessibility features.[9]

Until I was eight, my mum carried me to bed. In the grey-cladded house where I spent my early childhood, the only way to get to and from my bedroom as a disabled child was a piggyback. On the days my mum's back went, I would bump down the staircase on my bottom; a race to school punctuated with the singe of carpet. It was a game, although I know now of course it wasn't. I was lucky – in time, my family were able to move to a bungalow – but I quickly found that most other spaces were still closed off. Over the next thirty years, there hasn't been a single friend or family member's home that has been accessible to me. There are loved ones I have known for decades whose front room I've never seen and will never be able to. That is something that feels both staggering and completely unremarkable.

It is not as if life outside the home for disabled people is more welcoming. Just 15 per cent of restaurants and shops in the country have hearing loops,[10] while only 1 per cent of space at sporting venues is made available for disabled fans.[11] I have regularly sat for seven hours sipping one drink in a pub because there is no accessible toilet. I have missed a friend's wedding due to the fact the venue had no lift. I have sat outside restaurants eating in the cold because the website falsely said a wheelchair user could get inside. I would like to say there is outrage each time but, as I think we all know, nothing happens. At best, a manager emails a muted apology. Most of the time, no one says a thing. The lesson for disabled women comes early and it comes often:

the problem is not how society is built – the problem is your body.

It isn't only infrastructure we're shut out of – it's a decent income too. Disabled people are more likely than others to struggle for money; nearly half the people in poverty in the UK are disabled or live with a disabled person.[12] We are on average paid less than non-disabled people,[13] more likely to be turned down for a job[14] and less likely to be given senior roles at work,[15] all while shouldering the extra costs of disability[16] with often insufficient or no support from government benefits.[17]

On top of this, disabled people routinely face negative attitudes from the public. Some of these are openly hostile: that disabled people are lazy, faking, or burdens. Some are more benevolent but just as damaging, such as disabled people are vulnerable and need to be cared for or don't have the same intelligence, feelings or interests as other people. Research by the disability charity Scope in 2022[18] shows the scale of this: a quarter of disabled people had been accused of 'faking' their condition or not really being disabled, while a third had experienced people making assumptions about them or judging their capabilities based on their disability. This idea that disabled people are inherently different to 'normal people' is not a niche prejudice but startlingly common: separate research by Scope[19] shows over one in ten non-disabled people 'hardly ever' or 'never' think of disabled people as the same as everyone else. Even talking about disability is a taboo. Nearly half of the British public (45 per cent) admit to not feeling comfortable saying the word 'disabled' or 'disability' in everyday conversations.[20]

Growing up, I know all this shaped the way I saw myself and the life ahead of me. I surveyed a world around me that was not made for people like me, and worse, actively kept us out. As a child, I had no idea what it was to be a disabled woman, or that it was possible to be happy, have a career, or relationships. This only increased when I got sick. It's no wonder. Women are routinely fed the message that we must be perfect; that any hint of fallibility or difference – a career misstep, an anxious mind, a diet that includes gluten – means we are somehow failing. Disabled girls, meanwhile, are raised in a society that says disability is an inherently negative thing – the ultimate imperfection – and that it can never co-exist with love, talent, and fulfilment. Every open-mouthed stare at a club when you laugh from your wheelchair, every comment from a stranger that they would rather die than be like you, sends a painfully clear message about how life with a disability is 'meant' to be. We are taught from an early age that good health is the precursor to a positive existence, even more than wealth or social prestige. 'At least you've got your health!' the adage goes. But what if you haven't? It is hard to imagine the world has wonderful things to offer you when it routinely tells you it doesn't. We might call it the fog of low expectation, where society assumes a so-called broken body means a broken life – and the disabled women countering that stereotype are hidden from view.

This is not because there aren't many of us. Almost a quarter of people in the UK have some sort of disability – be it a physical impairment, mental health condition or chronic illness.[21] That's around 16 million people whose daily life is affected by a disability[22] – or the equivalent of the population of London twice over. That's a staggering number when you really stop to think about it. Look at the global picture and the scale is even more vast: the World Health Organization estimates there are 1.3 billion people globally who have 'significant disabilities'.[23]

What's more, the disabled club is not an exclusive one: any one of us can develop a long-term health condition at any point in our lives and find ourselves part of this community. That's even more the case if you're a woman. Women are more likely to have a long-term health condition than men,[24] with the World Health Survey estimating that the prevalence of disability among women is 60 per cent higher than our male counterparts.[25] The number of young women with disabilities in the UK is only increasing. One in seven women in their twenties are now classed as disabled as of 2023 – triple the previous figure – in part because the census for England and Wales now includes mental health in its question about disability.[26] Women are also disproportionately affected by a range of specific conditions, from depression,[27] autoimmune disorders[28] such as multiple sclerosis[29], to osteoporosis.[30] Disabled women are by far the biggest minority group in the world but we are still the least visible. Where are our voices? Why aren't we part of the conversation?

This doesn't mean we aren't contributing. Far from it. Disabled women are making waves like never before, ushering in societal change through politics, business, acting, science, sport, music, journalism, and more. Some of the most famous and influential women in the world today have a long-term health condition, from Greta Thunberg (autism), Billie Eilish (Tourette's), Greta Gerwig (ADHD), Selena Gomez (lupus and bipolar), to Lady Gaga (fibromyalgia). We are winning Oscars, leading communities, and legislating in parliaments. We are topping the charts, campaigning for equality, and winning gold medals. Imagine what it would be like if these stories were put front and centre of mainstream culture. Imagine what it would feel like if women's disabilities were not just acknowledged, but celebrated.

Over the last four years, I have spoken in-depth to fifty-plus incredible disabled women and non-binary people in order to do just that. Some have visible disabilities, others you may have watched on television and never known they had a hidden condition. Some have physical chronic illnesses, others are dealing with their mental health. Some were born with their disabilities, others fell ill later in life.

What they all share in common is this: they have blazed a trail in their fields, and done it all while sick or disabled. Throughout the pages of this book, they will talk candidly about anything, from careers, body confidence, to relationships. I spoke to Rosie Jones about what it's like to be on a dating app as a gay disabled woman, Ruth Madeley about missing months of school from surgeries, and Fearne Cotton on forging a career alongside her mental health. I chatted to Katie Piper about how she built confidence with her scars, Nikki Fox on learning to love her mobility aid, and Jameela Jamil about safe and fun sex with a disability.

These women and many more will not only share the challenges they have faced, but how they have jumped the same kind of barriers that sit in front of you. No one is going to pretend structural inequality isn't real – in fact, we will talk about it in detail – or that with enough willpower, disabled people can (or should) somehow overcome it. Instead, they will share the tools and strategies they've developed to navigate life as a disabled woman or non-binary person, and how doing things differently can be worn as a badge of pride. The purpose is not ever to downplay the difficulties that can come with disability or mental or physical illness but to show that happiness can – and does – run alongside it. This book will never claim to represent every experience (disability and health conditions are as varied as the millions of people with them) but with the help of these contributors, I'll do my best to show as many perspectives as possible.

Together, we will redefine what it is to be a woman with a disability today, and embrace every unique part. The mess, the joy and the pain.

This is not your typical book about disability. No one is going to get magically healed. There will be very little 'overcoming' anything. Years on from that night in the pub, I'm still sick. I'm still disabled. But I'm proud of my body, achieving, and laughing. Also occasionally weeping. This is not the narrative society is used to. They don't make Hallmark movies about someone never learning to walk again. But I think it is a much more important story. It is easy to be celebratory when you've made it to the top of the mountain, much harder when you're stuck halfway, freezing your tits off. One thing makes that mountain easier, though: knowing it's not just you on it. If there is any crumb that I hope you take away from the following pages, it is the feeling that there are many women in the world right now who are experiencing the same things you are. Because you're not alone in this. That's a promise.

On my more philosophical days, I think of bad health as something that naturally happens to living things. The pink peonies that brown at the edges. The honeybee that stings only to fall, depleted, through the air. Human beings are no different, really. We wilt. We go a little stale or pongy. The difference is, for us, it is not the end. The clocks don't stop. The music still plays. We go on. In a society that greets disability with low expectations or outright prejudice, and demands perfection from the mess of modern existence, I will share a secret: it is entirely possible to be happy and fulfilled and be disabled or sick, and to proudly carve out your own path. Who wants normal anyway?

School

'My headteacher just presumed that's what
happened to disabled children, that they
were institutionalized.'
— **Rt Hon. Marsha de Cordova MP**

When I was nine, I would race down the crisp aisle of Morrisons. I had got my first wheelchair only months earlier and the supermarket had become my training ground. Houses and classrooms were small and sticky with carpet, but this – *this* – was a place for adventure. I remember the smooth shine of the supermarket floor; freshly mopped laminate a perfect surface for spinning wheels. If I felt really wild, I would let loose down the wine aisle, neatly foreshadowing my early twenties.

I had needed a wheelchair long before this point in my childhood but had made do with a buggy; a plastic pile of hospital-grade seating, ugly and cumbersome. My new wheelchair was flash, streamlined and speedy. I adored the colour named 'Midnight Purple', as if the stars were flickering just for me.

In the hour after school, the supermarket became a regular haunt. My mum would occasionally allow me to pick a snack off the shelf, and I would eat along the way; perfecting wheelies in between nibbling Monster Munch. I would eventually emerge proudly from the aisle, a packet of crisps held in my hand a better trophy than any golden cup. At the till, I would watch the cashier scan the empty foil and smile at the thought of my secret adventures as it beeped.

The following year, I was almost big enough to leave primary school. Growing up in a small Lincolnshire town in the mid-90s, girls heading to secondary education had one of two main options: the state grammar or the all-girls comprehensive in a step-filled tower block. The latter didn't exactly seem a practical option for me. I imagined myself doing physics stuck at the bottom of the tower, a kind of Rapunzel in reverse. My wheelchair, which in the crisp aisle had brought me such freedom, at school seemed to mean limitation.

Luckily, I passed my 11+. It turns out, though, that this wasn't enough if you were disabled, as it so rarely tends to be. No one who used a wheelchair had ever been to the grammar school before, which meant no one had bothered to make it accessible. It may not have been a tower block, but it might as well have been: a rabbit warren of carpeted stairs and corridors to nowhere. It meant that in Year 7, my form had all our classes taught out of two rooms – because

2

they were the only ones I could get into. The downstairs English room became both an English room and a maths room. And a geography room. And an everything-else room. I was relieved to learn it wasn't also the accessible toilet.

Over the years, my school slowly opened up to me: a lift down to the dining hall, then one to modern languages, another upstairs to history, and finally a ramp for the sixth-form common room. It was glacial access, akin to a DIY SOS if the crew had got distracted halfway through. I was lucky. I got used to fighting and had the support to do it. I had parents who would go in to bat for me. I had a kind headteacher. But looking back, it is strange to feel 'lucky' to have been allowed to go to school. Life was only just starting and the message was loud and clear: disabled girls can't have what everyone else has.

I didn't realize it at the time but what I was experiencing with my wheelchair was what many disabled teenagers go through every day. There are countless barriers for us just to access school like other pupils, whether that's steps into classrooms, lack of British Sign Language teaching assistants, or inadequate mental health support. Disabled girls can face hurdles at every stage of their education, from the lack of physical access, low expectations of teachers, to juggling coursework with time off sick. It turns out that getting in the building is only the beginning.

D is (not) for disability

Every summer on exam results day, my local paper would feature pupils from my school who had excelled. It was the coveted spot of success: a row of grinning girls who had got straight As, spread over a black and white page. Through the years, I never saw a disabled girl make that photo.[*] When it came to my own GCSE results day, I wouldn't say I was optimistic – more nauseous with a hint of hysteria. It wasn't that I hadn't revised. Every exam morning, I would get up at 5 a.m. to cram, reading over note cards in the dark that I had already scanned a hundred times. It never struck me that this was an unusual effort or bordering on overkill. Working around the clock felt an entirely rational response to disability. I understood early on that someone who had a body like mine could not be average. I wanted things that I was not supposed to. A top university place. A fulfilling career. And I knew that to get them, I was going to have to work harder than most other people. When someone assumed my disability meant I wasn't capable or intelligent, I would have a piece of paper to prove otherwise. I suppose this only increased the pressure I felt over exams. Disabled girls can't afford to make mistakes.

---

[*] There could of course have been someone who had an invisible disability. It's interesting how the fact many health conditions aren't visible impacts not only how non-disabled people see us but how we see ourselves. We'll come back to that.

I remember waking up on results morning and grabbing the first thing I found to wear – a crinkly sky-blue top that resembled old pyjamas. When I got to school, I noticed my deputy headteacher smiling unnervingly from the back of the hall. A petite woman who had gone grey young, she raced towards me, as if I had won the lottery. Disappointingly, I had not won a cash prize but I had scored 100 per cent in my GCSE English literature. Ushered towards the photographer from the paper, I tried to quickly get a grip. I looked like I had just rolled out of bed, because I had. I remember the inane quote I gave to the reporter: 'I didn't even think it had gone well.' I don't think my shock was purely down to my disability but it certainly played a part. I had never seen anyone achieve who looked like me. It didn't occur to me it was possible.

When the media discusses education and success, we get one recurring image: white, pretty non-disabled girls, often found spontaneously jumping in the air on exam results day. At the other end of the spectrum, we hear of struggling 'white working-class boys' or the problem of 'excluded black boys', often with clearly racist undertones. We hear very little of disabled pupils, and even less about disabled girls. It can feel like society doesn't think much at all about disabled young people, and when they do, that they don't have high hopes for us. Culturally, disability is still often associated with tragedy, helplessness, and an inability to think for ourselves.

It means that it is too often assumed that pupils with disabilities and health conditions don't have the same talents, interests and goals as everyone else. The truth is, mainstream culture often doesn't acknowledge disabled young people even exist in the first place. When much of the general public think of 'disability', they tend to imagine an older, frail person. Or to put it another way: they are more likely to picture a nan in a nursing home than a fifteen-year-old in French class. It is true that people often acquire a disability as they get older but many of us have a physical or mental health condition from a young age. Almost one in ten children in the UK have a disability of some sort.[1] How are they doing? What qualifications are they getting?

There's a noticeable lack of research on the attainment of disabled pupils but from what is available, the picture is pretty stark: teenagers with disabilities consistently struggle to get the same sort of grades as their peers. Research by the University of Warwick and the London School of Economics in 2018[2] found the problems start early, with disabled children more likely to leave primary school and enter secondary education with lower educational attainment than non-disabled pupils. The study found this continued throughout school life, resulting in disabled pupils being significantly less likely to achieve good grades at GCSE: a minuscule 26 per cent achieve five or more grades at A*–C, including English and maths, compared to 67 per cent of non-disabled students. Research also shows that disabled young people are more likely to leave school without passing any exams at all. The Office for National Statistics (ONS) shows 15 per cent of disabled people in the UK have no qualifications[3] compared with just 5 per cent of non-disabled people.[4]

Even those disabled pupils who do manage to excel often end up missing out on the same opportunities as their non-disabled peers. The University of Warwick found that the 26 per cent of young people with disabilities who achieve five or more A*–C grades are less likely to stay on to take A levels than young people without disabilities.[5] Only 75 per cent of disabled students who have done well at GCSE continue in full-time upper-secondary education, compared to 85 per cent of non-disabled students.

Screenwriter and actor Genevieve Barr, who is deaf,* knows this first-hand. While Barr managed academically at school, lack of official support meant she had to jump multiple hurdles compared to her non-disabled peers to get there. 'In many ways, I had a great time at school. I got good grades and was a bit of a sports nut. I had a riotous group of friends and I milked my hearing aids for every advantage I could get away with. But looking back, there is stuff I tried to forget – being left out of primary-school sports teams and plays, being forced to sit and listen to the radio

---

* Throughout this book, you'll see I capitalize the word 'Deaf' but sometimes use lower-case 'deaf' to describe contributors. This is to respect the choice of how they wish to identify.

7

every week, the lack of subtitles for every video. I remember feeling lonely because sometimes I wanted a friend who was deaf like me, who understood how tiring it is to lip-read. I didn't have a teaching assistant or an educational statement and there were definitely times when I was expected to just "get on with it". One particular teacher liked to have us write down verbatim what he said for whole lessons. When that happened, my classmates would let me read over their shoulder and I would copy what they were writing into my own book. When I got caught looking in any other direction than the teacher, I got scolded. They knew I wasn't lip-reading them.'

I was a teenager when I was first patted on the head by a stranger, like a human Labrador. From a young age, many of us with a visible disability will have had these encounters. Members of the public speaking incredibly loudly for no reason. Shop assistants talking to the non-disabled person next to you. Asking for the bill in a restaurant only to have the receipt handed to your non-disabled date. These individuals are not acting this way to everyone they meet, of course. They are doing it specifically to disabled people. They are doing it because they believe that having a disability makes us less capable than other, 'normal' people.

This behaviour isn't just a small annoyance. It's an exaggerated version of the patronizing attitudes that directly impact why some disabled girls struggle to fulfil their potential at school – and, moreover, why society is less likely to do anything about it. If you think disability means a teenager can't be bright or hardworking, it's natural to believe the disability attainment gap exists because we just aren't clever enough to do well at school. If you assume disabled pupils don't have the same goals or ambitions as their non-disabled peers, it's easy not to worry when they start falling behind.

In reality, poor attainment of disabled pupils is in no way inherently linked with our disability or health conditions. Instead, it's down to a complex web of social and environmental factors. Dr Sarah Chave, an affiliate to the University of Exeter, who researches education and disability and who herself has an inflammatory condition, says: 'Despite many years of campaigning and legislation aiming to prevent discrimination, disabled pupils still face barriers at school and college. These barriers impact disabled students' wellbeing and educational achievement.

'The barriers can be physical, such as inaccessible classrooms, toilets or libraries. For example, stairs and narrow doorways block pupils who use wheelchairs, badly lit corridors can be a problem for visually impaired students, or a lack of hearing-loop systems can create barriers for hearing-impaired students. Lack of quiet spaces to rest creates barriers for students who need places to recuperate mentally and physically during the busy and loud school day.

'But it's also social attitudes and culture, things like teacher attitude and not being included, lack of disabled teachers, and attitudes of classmates towards their disabled peers and loneliness that can come with that. Teachers often have inadequate training about disabilities and how these impact students. There are significantly few teachers with disabilities, which both creates a lack of role models for disabled students and also makes it difficult for teachers to learn from one another about disability.'

In many ways, this generation of disabled pupils are benefiting from considerable progress in how schools understand and address disability. Only several decades ago, it was normal for disabled young people to be segregated in 'special schools' away from other children or given no real education at all. Nowadays, most of us are rightly schooled alongside our non-disabled peers and are – on paper at least – given similar opportunities to our classmates. But as Chave explains, despite this progress, disabled pupils are still at a severe disadvantage. This has only been exacerbated in recent years when the UK has seen some support services rolled back, with experts warning funding cuts are causing a 'full-blown crisis' in special needs education.[6] Forget dream A-level results – for thousands of disabled pupils, they don't even have a school place.[7] Others have had their specialist support worker removed; four out of five headteachers[8] have been forced to cut back on teaching assistants in recent years, while one in ten teachers of the Deaf have been cut.[9]

With the right support and access arrangements in place, pupils with disabilities and health conditions have every chance to fulfil their potential on an equal footing to our peers. Take it away, and it's no wonder we struggle. As Chave puts it: '[Prejudice around disability] leads to a culture where disabled pupils are too often framed as the "problem" to be fixed. In fact, it's social and environmental factors which disable pupils rather than any so-called "impairments". If schools were to address these, more and more pupils could feel pride in their disabilities and thrive in education.'

One of my biggest barriers at school was that I wasn't always able to be there. A weak immune system combined with the fact children are germ factories meant chunks of the winter term were often spent in bed with a chest infection. I had got myself into a routine of sorts: catch a bug, spend a few weeks ill at home, go back to school for a while, then catch another. I had kind teachers, several of whom went the extra mile for me, but I was often expected to catch up by myself. I remember returning to school after one particular absence and being given only one strategy to learn what I'd missed: a maths textbook to flick through while everyone else did PE. I thought this was entirely normal. I'd always been pretty good at maths – by the end of primary school, I was in the year above for arithmetic – but as I got older, and the workload increased, things got more difficult. By the time I was fifteen, my catch-up method largely involved watching *Countdown*. In the end, I scraped by with a C in GCSE maths and was relieved to manage that. To this day, I cannot comprehend algebra but can recognize Carol Vorderman with one eye shut.

I'm far from alone in this. A study by the disability charity Mind in 2021[10] found nearly seven in ten young people reported being absent from school due to their mental health. In some cases, this resulted in them falling out of education altogether. There is no comparable study of young people with physical disabilities, but anecdotally, it's an issue that affects many of us. The school system is not built for young people who need to take time off. Teachers drill into us that skipping class is skiving. Many schools even give out attendance awards; a chocolate cup for the victory of not getting sick. Meanwhile, pupils who do fall ill are often discouraged from convalescing. In 2024, the UK government launched a campaign[11] to urge parents to send their children to school despite having cold symptoms or stomach aches, with some parents of children who have long-term health conditions even being prosecuted for truancy.[12] Overall, it's a system that too often rewards pupils for the luck of good health and marginalizes those without it.

Actor Ruth Madeley can identify with this. Born with spina bifida, she missed a year and a half of school in-person due to needing multiple surgeries on her spine as a teenager. In the end, she completed her GCSE coursework from bed. 'I really enjoyed school and I had a really good group of friends [but I missed quite a bit of class time]. My grades were always pretty good so I put a lot of pressure on myself to do well, especially when I had to miss a lot of school due to spinal surgeries. I had great teachers, except one maths teacher who wasn't particularly good at helping me with work when I was in hospital. [It meant] my parents [had to get] me a maths tutor to help prepare me for my GCSEs. Maths was never my favourite subject and was the one subject I worried about the most, so I felt even worse having to catch up after spending so much time in hospital in the build-up to my GCSEs. Getting a tutor helped me so much but I know how privileged I was to have one.'

Jameela Jamil, an actor and activist who has the connective tissue condition Ehlers–Danlos syndrome (EDS), experienced a similar lack of support. 'I spent a large portion of my childhood and teens in bed due to EDS and how clumsy it makes you and how long it takes to heal when you get hurt. I was always having to fight to catch up as I was constantly behind the others, so I would say I was permanently stressed from the age of six to seventeen! It was a true bore. It was also so isolating being so different from other kids, and missing key moments and development, so I was fairly lonely because of it. My school were not supportive and threatened at one point to expel me for time missed through illness. The pressure to keep up with my very non-disabled classmates was hell without any extra support.'

After being in a car accident and facing injuries on top of her disability, the lack of help from her school led Jamil to drop out. 'When I was hit by the car, I still had my A levels to do, and after a year and a half of TV, ice cream and morphine, I was offered my scholarship back, and frankly could not be fucked to go back to a life of desperately catching up again. So, I just left school and started getting odd jobs. I abandoned my dream of working in medicine and just wanted to live in the real world. I was so grateful to be able to walk again that I was just desperate to see, eat and experience everything (apart from anal, I am extremely precious about my bumhole).'

A few weeks after I had written what I thought was the final word of this chapter, a shocking headline flashed up on my phone: disabled children had been 'erased' from their class photo in a primary school in Aberdeenshire.[13] In early 2024, a photographer is said to have taken separate pictures: one with the pupils with 'additional needs' and one without. Parents were then given both versions to choose from. Reportedly, a set of twins were split up. The child who uses a wheelchair was excluded from one photo, while their twin without a disability was photographed with the rest of their class.

It was a bleak and particularly blatant window into how bigotry towards disabled children festers, how the prejudice around disability that I had been worrying about – that it is lesser, abnormal, a fault best erased – can mould our young lives before we even leave the classroom.

In this context, it's not hard to imagine that – on top of the practical barriers we've discussed so far – these kind of social factors affect whether disabled pupils can flourish at school. Take perceptions about disability. There's research to suggest that concerns about the future actively influence how high disabled pupils aim while at school. A study by the University of Warwick[14] into why disabled pupils did not carry on with formal education found the biggest influence was actually educational expectations – both the expectations of the young people themselves, and those of others. It found disabled young people were 15 percentage points more likely to have low expectations about going to university than non-disabled students of similar backgrounds. Interestingly, their hopes about their future were still muted when they were getting good grades; the research discovered that even when disabled pupils are achieving academically at similar levels to their non-disabled peers, there remained a 10 percentage point gap in expectations.

This is hardly surprising. For any young person, it can be daunting at fourteen to predict what shape your life will take at thirty-four. But growing up with a health condition, this can be all the tougher. If your fatigue is fluctuating, it can be difficult to know what your body will be able to do in a month's time, let alone a few decades. If adults around you are treating you differently than your non-disabled peers, it can be hard to dare dream the same. This is only compounded by the fact there is still a lack of visible role models for aspiring disabled teenagers, even down to the materials used in job fairs. When I was at school, spotting a disabled woman in a career poster in my sixth-form common room was like completing a particularly advanced *Where's Wally?* book ('he's hiding near the back, between the unemployment line and my hopes of being a homeowner by the time I hit menopause'). It's not easy to picture yourself as a solicitor or doctor when you've never seen one who looks like you. I'll talk more about the power of representation in a later chapter, but for now I will say this: we do not show disabled girls a world where we value the thoughts and brains of disabled women. We do not show those struggling in their teens that adulthood can bring wonders. This can all make it seem as if there are a narrow range of possibilities for young disabled women's futures, even when there are a host of opportunities for fulfilling courses and careers. Or to put it another way: exclusion does not need to be as explicit as a photographer asking the disabled pupils to leave the room. Often, it is just the unspoken suggestion that we simply don't belong there.

Indeed, low expectations aren't just an issue of how disabled pupils see themselves – it's their teachers and parents too. The same Warwick study[15] found parents of disabled young people tend to have lower educational expectations for them due to fears about university or job prospects, something that remains regardless of their actual achievement. It is a kind of self-fulfilling prophecy, where concern over low opportunities and success for disabled young people leads them to take fewer chances to succeed.

Dr Stella Chatzitheochari, who was part of the research team at the University of Warwick, says: 'Our research found that parents' expectations were lower for disabled young people, regardless of their actual performance. This leads to a situation where disabled young people have lower educational and occupational expectations than their non-disabled peers, even when they attain as well in school. Parents of disabled young people are generally quite "protective" in an attempt to shield young people from future disappointment. This may be because they are expecting discrimination in the labour market or lack of support for their disabilities in higher education.

'It's [a kind of loving response] to the difficulties they see facing their children. I've spoken to parents whose children had done well at school and went to university but were unable to get a job later due to their disability, who told me they felt guilty they hadn't prepared them for this. Likewise, I've spoken to parents who said, "We don't want to get her hopes up, we know how hard it is out there."'

There's minimal research in this area but it's clear that expectations of teachers can be a problem too. When I studied for my A levels, I was fortunate to be predicted three As and have an interview lined up for Cambridge. I had several supportive teachers but years later, I still remember the two who suggested I apply for universities that were ranked significantly lower. There was nothing wrong with the courses – league tables don't define how much we prosper at uni – but it felt like they were setting the bar low for me. I couldn't imagine those teachers talking to my non-disabled classmates who had similar grades and advising them to dream smaller.

Dr Angharad Butler-Rees, a postdoctoral researcher at the University of Warwick, who herself is visually impaired, has conducted multiple studies into the school life of disabled pupils and has found the attitudes of teachers to be a factor in why students with disabilities may struggle. 'From speaking to young disabled people as part of our research, many have told us how they feel teachers have lower aspirations for them than their peers. This might be because some teachers have had little prior interaction with disabled people or have little awareness or understanding of disability. Teachers' low expectations of students, and outright prejudice, can have a big impact on their grades. For example, it prevents them from being put in higher classroom sets or being put forward for higher-tier exam papers. [It's a catch-22]: teachers may assume that disabled young people are less capable of achieving higher grades due to their disability, and that means disabled young people can end up not getting the opportunities and support needed to get higher grades.'

Samantha Renke, a broadcaster and disability consult-ant who has a brittle bone condition, found a mix of both physical access and social attitudes affected her chances at school. 'My primary school was linked to a high school which meant that all the kids bar a few exceptions would automat-ically go there. But it was a very old building and it needed ramps and lifts to be accessible. They seemed happy to adapt it but as time went on, it was suggested the building was "too old" to "meet my needs", money being the key factor. I remember someone said that the school had recently gotten stained-glass windows replaced but apparently they couldn't afford disability access. That has always stayed with me.'

It meant Renke had to attend another school just because it was one she could physically get into. 'I knew no one at the school as my friends had gone to the other, inaccessible one, and I became "that kid in the wheelchair". I had a teaching assistant but would have to wait for her to finish her lunch before I could go out and play and even then everyone was on edge just in case someone would bang into me and break a bone. I spent most of my lunchtimes hanging out in the disabled toilet. Glamorous! Academically, I feel like I underachieved – a few Bs, Cs, Ds at GCSE and one A. I spent a lot of my time trying to fit in, trying to get people to like me, rather than concentrate on my studies. At the time, my mindset was more "survive today" – the next operation, where to get the next funding for my wheelchair – instead of thinking about tomorrow. I remember a conversation in primary school with one teacher, when the subject of what do you want to be when you grow up was asked. Without hesitation I said, "Well I need to go to high school, college, university, and I want to be an actress or if not an actress a teacher." The teacher just smiled in a dismissive "OK, we'll see". Ironically, that's the exact path I took.'

As a Member of Parliament and former Shadow Secretary of State, the Rt Hon. Marsha de Cordova MP, who is visually impaired, has held one of the highest offices in the country. But as a child, the low expectations of teachers meant she was almost denied a mainstream education altogether. 'Education was a bumpy start for me. At primary school, the then headteacher thought that I should be moved to a "special school" due to my visual impairment. There was an assumption I wouldn't be as capable as a non-disabled pupil or didn't need the same education. I think there was also an element of just not wanting to provide support for me, and also the fact my headteacher just presumed that's what happened to disabled children, that they were institutionalized. I was made by the school to undergo various assessments, but my mum fought for me to remain in mainstream education. I ended up staying at my primary school and then going to a mainstream secondary school, where I was given support. I'm so grateful for my mum. Without that decision, I wouldn't be where I am today.'

Having non-disabled people fight alongside us like this can significantly ease the load for disabled pupils. This allyship can take many simple forms. If you're a teacher, you could check your unconscious bias and consider if you're treating your disabled pupils in the same way as the rest of your class. If you're a student attending an after-school activity, you might ask the organizers if it's accessible for a range of disabilities. If you're a caregiver or parent to a non-disabled child, you could talk to them early on about disability and normalize this aspect of the friends they might go on to meet. Disability is as much a part of school life as homework and inedible lunches. Looking out for your disabled classmates and students can make a genuine difference.

'Growing up with cerebral palsy, which affects my speech and movement . . . I'd get the odd poor teacher who would say, "No, Rosie, you can't read out, it would take too long,"' says Rosie Jones, a comedian and television presenter. 'If any teachers would stop me from doing something, I would always call them out on it, question it, and challenge their ableism. It definitely took much more confidence and self-assurance to stand up to teachers who patronized or underestimated me [than it did other children]. But luckily, I had the best parents who would always fight in my corner and help me achieve my full potential . . . [They] told me that I could be whoever I wanted to be. Apart from a hairdresser.

'In the best possible way, I was a very arrogant child, but that is the way I *had* to be in order to make school work for me . . . Growing up with a disability made me stubborn, determined and ambitious. If anybody suggested that I couldn't do something, I would go out of my way to prove them wrong. It made me the strong-willed nightmare of a woman I am today and I wouldn't have it any other way.'

Just like with adults, Jones found herself facing a few class-mates who belittled her. '"Get some fucking proper legs!" That's a remark that particularly stands out to me from my school years. I remember not feeling sad, or angry. I think I was fifteen and the boy who yelled it at me from across the school car park was three years younger than me. I actually remember feeling quite sorry for the boy. I thought it was funny that he waited until I was a good ten feet away from him, as if he was scared of me, and my response. And I remember thinking that the comment was just ridiculous. Where would I get some fucking proper legs from? A fucking proper leg shop? The boy was shouting utter nonsense at me.

'I was always so confident in my own skin I think it was almost impossible to bully me. I'd just always agree with them, or shrug it off . . . An idiot would say my walk was stupid, to which I would answer, "Yes, it is, but I like it." I always knew that their comments came from an unhappi-ness or anger within themselves, and often it wasn't to do with me at all.'

Jones counts herself as lucky – 'I think I got called the "R word" once in all my time at school,' she says – but bullying can be another significant factor in why disabled pupils can struggle in education. Large-scale *Lancet* research in 2022, which reviewed over ninety studies across 16 million children in twenty-five countries, found almost 40 per cent of disabled children globally experienced bullying by their peers. Things aren't much better here. Research *Doubly Disadvantaged*, published in the *Sage Journal* in 2015,[16] shows that, by age seven, pupils with special needs are twice as likely to be bullied than those without disabilities. By the age of fifteen, disabled teenagers are at a higher risk of being excluded from friendship groups, while all school-age children are more likely to be bullied 'all the time' than their non-disabled peers. For a generation who grew up online, social media can magnify this: as well as 'in-person' abuse, the study found disabled young people are also more likely to be victims of cyberbullying, such as classmates sharing 'embarrassing' photos and spreading rumours online. All of this naturally has a significant impact not only on whether disabled pupils have the chance to get good grades, but on their mental health and how much they can enjoy school.

Lucy Webster, a journalist who has cerebral palsy and uses a wheelchair, can relate to these findings. 'I went to a private girls' school – the local council had no answer for what to do with a bright disabled kid – which had the unintended effect that [my peers] were very clever about bullying,' she says. 'No one ever said anything that could have got them in trouble, but they would do things like invite me to lunch and then sit where I couldn't get in my chair, or make sure

I knew about parties I wasn't invited to. It was an extreme form of ostracization, made infinitely worse by the fact they would be nice to me, at random, when it suited them. Looking back, I was fairly depressed between the ages of twelve and eighteen . . . I spent a lot of mornings in tears, trying to get out of going to school, and I can still feel the knot of anxiety I had in my stomach for most of the time.

'I was the only visibly disabled person in the school and (I think) the only wheelchair user they'd ever had . . . I think the school had no idea what to do with me – they assumed "equality" meant treating me exactly the same as everyone else, and extended this approach beyond all reason, like making me play lacrosse! They were in complete denial about the fact I was different, which only served to put me in more positions where that difference became a problem, which really only gave the bullies more ammunition. I felt as if I stuck out like a sore thumb, which I think drove me to try to fit in or conform. I tried not talking about disability, not asking for help, not saying no to things I couldn't do and generally pretending everything was fine when it really wasn't. It wasn't mentally healthy and it wasn't successful either.'

As one of the only learning disabled girls in her secondary school, model Ellie Goldstein, who has Down's syndrome, was picked on because she looked different. 'Growing up, I was always aware that I was shorter than my friends and older girls sometimes used to make fun of that.

They would say, "Why are you so little?" They didn't know it was just part of having Down's syndrome. Sometimes the questions were curiosity but sometimes it wasn't said in a nice way. I went to mainstream primary school and mainstream secondary school until Year 10 when I moved to a mild/moderate special needs school to complete my exams, so being one of the only pupils with a disability made others notice that I looked different than the other girls. It made me notice it too. I was the only one with a scar down my chest to my stomach from my open-heart surgery when I was five months old, so I felt different. I always stood up for myself, though, and didn't take any notice of others saying things to me. My parents made me feel confident and brought me up like my sister and not with the disability first. That always helped me feel secure in myself, even if I had trouble with other girls.'

Butler-Rees says this is a common experience for disabled young women. 'Finding a welcoming and supportive group of friends at school can be a challenge for any student. But from my research, I've found these relationships are particularly valued by disabled girls. [Those] I've interviewed often struggled with their identity, feeling uncomfortable in themselves and taking a long time to understand and embrace [who they are]. Some girls also found it difficult to find a peer group where they could be accepted. Disabled girls, for example, often spoke of trying to hide or mask their impairments so as to "fit in" with their friends, something that I myself remember doing as a disabled pupil. While hiding or masking your disability is exhausting, it can also make it harder for disabled girls to receive the right support at school. Teachers may be unaware that the young person is struggling or would benefit from additional support, such as alternative exam arrangements. That all inevitably prevents disabled pupils achieving their full potential.'

'Trying to fit in' is one of those impulses that is notorious during our teenage years, but as Butler-Rees says, it can be all the more palpable for those of us with a disability, and can stay with us years after we leave school. If you're the only disabled girl in your class, it's natural to feel as if you stick out sometimes, like a zebra in an enclosure of sheep. Maybe you're going through this at the moment. Maybe your schooldays are long behind you, but the memory still niggles at your gut. In a world that too often tells you that what you are isn't good enough, at a time in your life when you're full of self-doubt, let me tell you this: you are under no obligation to conform with your classmates, have no duty to be anything but your wonderful disabled self. You are just as smart and full of brilliance as anyone without a disability – hell, with all you're coping with, I bet you've got more skills and strength than most. I hope the disabled women sharing their hurdles over the past few pages can teach one particularly important lesson: your schooldays do not determine the rest of your life. If things are hard right now, hold on. It is more than possible to be crying in your bedroom when you're fifteen and laughing with friends at twenty-five. This is just the beginning for you. There are a thousand adventures ahead.

Growing pains

I have spent several pages extolling the virtues of disabled pupils having the chance to get good grades. Let me now do something that would score a D in any essay: a sudden and dramatic U-turn.

It is OK to fail your exams. It is OK to be overwhelmed and crash out of formal education entirely. It is OK to sit in your dressing gown watching *This Morning* and scream: 'IT'S CALLED THE UNIVERSITY OF LIFE, OK?' You deserve to be given every bit of support necessary for the best shot at school: be it extra time in exams, help during absences, or adaptations in class. But the reality of disability means that sometimes – despite every bit of support, despite all our effort – we still might struggle to hit the same targets as our non-disabled friends.

It is natural to feel like exam results and 'achievement' are the be-all and end-all of life, or to dismiss the everyday wins of surviving a dodgy body. They don't invite you to study at Oxford because you managed to put a bra on this morning. Many of us go through life with the background belief that our accomplishments somehow define us, that we must earn our right to exist by meeting a certain standard of success at work or relationships – and first off, school. But

this mindset is rarely accurate and can be outright debilitating. Research by Mind in 2021 found many young people
reported that the pressure to succeed academically went
as far as to affect their mental health. Almost one in four
said school had made their mental health worse,[17] with
pupils expressing particular concern over the pressure to
do well in exams. Studies don't show the specific impact on
pupils who already had disabilities and health conditions
but it's not a stretch to imagine the pressure could be even
higher for us. Growing up throws up plenty of hassles to
deal with, from first relationships, exam anxiety, to regret-
table haircuts. If you're disabled, it just so happens you've
got extra. Hospital appointments. Long spells of time off
school. Not to mention the health symptoms themselves.
For disabled pupils, there's more to think about than
getting our coursework in.

While her classmates were focused on revising for
their GCSEs, Evie Torrance was dealing with debilitating glandular fever and doing her exams 'at home in my
pyjamas, with my head of year coming over to my house to
invigilate'. By the time of her AS levels, Torrance – now a
chronic-illness content creator and author – had developed
ME, Lyme disease and migraines and was forced to leave
school entirely. 'It's definitely affected my self-esteem. As I
became more ill that first year after dropping out of school, I
had to watch all my friends move on with their lives – going
off to university, travelling, becoming independent. I craved
these things so much that I got lost on what I didn't have

rather than what I did. [When I went out, the] small-talk questions of "What do you do for a living?" or "Where and what are you studying?" were constant. I actually used to lie to strangers. I used to tell them I was at Bristol studying psychology as I was too ashamed to admit I was a nineteen-year-old disabled person living at home with my parents.'

Ironically, it was when Torrance became housebound at twenty that she felt this pressure ease. 'It meant that for the first time, I no longer had to contend with questions of what I was doing with my life. I started to learn that my lack of qualifications didn't mean I was worth less. It wasn't something I learned overnight . . . But I'm no longer ashamed of my story. I'm no longer ashamed of my lack of qualifications. I know now that just because I can do less doesn't mean I'm worth less. Just because I'm a disabled adult living at home doesn't mean I'm not clever or ambitious. And just because my peers are doing things that externally appear to be more successful doesn't necessarily mean they are.

'Being pushed off the traditional education route can be absolutely terrifying, but it can push you to find what you love. At school, English was my worst subject, and I had to work really, *really* hard to get my A at GCSE. But one day, a few months after becoming housebound, I decided to start a blog. And my love of writing started there, and four years later, I self-published my first poetry and prose book. I know without a doubt that if I hadn't become ill, I would never have found my love of writing. I had to get pushed into the unknown first before I thought about "alternative" choices.'

Nowadays, Mollie Goodfellow is a screenwriter for hit television shows, but at school, mental health problems meant she missed out on her first plan of going to university. 'I'd been struggling with depression and anxiety for a while before starting sixth form, and ended up with some distinctly average A levels. At the end of sixth form, I also got myself one of those terrible teenage boyfriends who are just the absolute worst. He dumped me just before I was supposed to go to university and I just fully had a breakdown. Not just about him, about a lot of things. I was quite unwell and felt quite unsafe and was having some really dark thoughts and plans about suicide. I ended up in hospital and having some more intense therapy after that. I [was due to start] university to study fashion about a week after I left hospital [but] it just absolutely didn't feel right or safe at all, so I withdrew from my place and focused on getting well again. It felt quite strange for a while. The rest of my close friendship group all went to universities across the country. They were doing Freshers' Week and starting this next chapter of their lives and I was still in my parents' house crying about being sad.

'About six or eight months after I'd been really unwell, things started to turn around. I started writing my own blogs and eventually I got a job in social media. I then got myself a journalism apprenticeship at the *Evening Standard* and *Independent* newspapers, which luckily was only open to non-graduates, and in the end I got one of three jobs out of six hundred people. It really made me feel like I hadn't made a mistake with not pursuing university and that I wouldn't be treading water for the rest of my life. Within a year of working at that apprenticeship I'd written stories that were featured on the front page and was interviewing celebrities I'd only ever seen on TV. It was really magic. I've now started writing for television, which is an absolute dream. I'm hoping one day to write my own sitcom and have got a pilot in early development stages . . . I'm still working on my mental health to this day [but] I have no regrets about [how university turned out]. I really like who I am now and where I am now.'

I'm not going to pretend there is a point to health problems. That there is some grand plan for what you're going through. As Torrance and Goodfellow show, it is entirely possible that experiencing illness or disability will lead to growth or new opportunities, like pulling a rose from the dirt. Maybe growing up with a disability makes us more resilient than our peers. Maybe missing out on the traditional path of education leads to another, better road. But it is OK if things don't feel quite that serendipitous right now (and in the moment, I think it rarely does). 'Everything happens for a reason' is a comforting mantra but more comforting if what's happening is diamonds and great sex rather than morphine and incontinence pads. I reject the idea that there is a purpose to suffering. I reject the pressure to never feel heartbroken about the things we can't do. It simultaneously minimizes the pain that you're going through, while burdening you with the duty to see past it. When you think about it, it's pretty rude to suggest being disabled gives you an obligation to learn some sort of lesson, especially when you're barely out of school. No one would see a car crash and ask the passengers for the meaning of life. Still, I know that I am different than I would have been if I had been born with better genetics, just as I am different now I'm chronically ill than if I hadn't gone to the pub and caught flu that night. For all the loss and missed opportunities that health problems can bring, I have seen and survived things that most people my age could never imagine. You probably have too. It comes with a particular type of wisdom, like we are seeing an edge of the human experience that others just aren't aware of. It is as if I have travelled back from the future and can tell the church elders the earth is not flat after all.

One lesson falling ill young teaches you, I think, is that life does not always go to plan. A white shirt will inevitably get a red splodge of ketchup down it, your joints might pick the day of your university interview to flare up in pain. It's completely natural to find this frustrating, to want to have a cry under the bedsheets or eat your body weight in Doritos. Do all of the above if it helps. Cry. Become a human tortilla chip. But be kind to yourself too. There is a pleasure in deciding what sort of person you want to be. In seeing the limits that society has set for you and saying, '*No, thank you.*' But there is also something pretty remarkable about accepting your current boundaries. In struggling. In smack-down-on-your-face failing. And saying, 'This is not the end of the world.'

As disabled women, our path to achieving our goals might take a few detours – or the destination may change entirely. That's fine. You are not in competition with your non-disabled peers, nor a hypothetical healthy version of yourself. 'Success' takes more forms than the limited shape they tell you, and the biggest achievement can simply be getting through today. The cultural myth that the two years between our sixteenth and eighteenth birthdays is our only shot to determine our whole lives is preposterous, really, much like the idea that the only place we will get an education is the formal setting of a classroom. Life is long and full of opportunities, and there is so much more to you than the grade on an exam slip. If you miss your first chance, there will always be a second. Probably a forty-seventh.

As this chapter has shown, school life still poses obstacles for students with disabilities and health conditions: from the bias held by some teachers towards disabled pupils, inaccessible buildings, to a lack of practical measures like teaching assistants and providing tutoring during absences. Similarly, there may be times when our health means disabled young people will need to step off the traditional education path and go their own way. But we have also seen that with the right accommodations, disabled students can flourish at school or embrace the many opportunities that exist outside it.

When your formative years are spent fighting to access the same spaces as everyone else, it can be easy to feel there's something wrong with you. That if only your body could go faster or your mind worked differently, things would be so much easier. It took me a while to realize that isn't actually how this story goes. The reason I couldn't access those classrooms when I was eleven wasn't because my legs failed to walk but because no adult had thought to install a ramp. Twenty-five years on from the crisp aisle, I understand my wheelchair was never the problem – it was that the education system wasn't built for it. It should have been. And it should be built for you too.

University

'I was a different person at eighteen. Unsure of myself . . .
I should've put my foot down and said, "Tough shit, you
need to make me a disabled bay outside my flat."
But I didn't and that walk to the car park meant
I often didn't get to go to my classes.'
— **Nikki Fox**

One of my earliest memories is standing in the back garden of my grandparents' old council house, surveying two pigeons. Born in Ireland and a professional jockey in his youth, my granddad had turned to keeping homing pigeons – bred for speed and distance – as a little piece of his former life. Somewhere along the way, he had decided to name two of the pigeons after his infant granddaughters, perhaps the ultimate compliment.

In the fresh wind of rural Leicestershire, my elder sister and I found ourselves outside for a special occasion: our namesake pigeons were going to be released. Stocky creatures, the rival birds cooed in their box, their muted silver feathers flapping against the sides. Homing pigeons, by definition, are made for a particular type of journey: they may travel for hundreds of miles, but in time, they will find their way back home. We watched them fly into the sky that day, not knowing when they would return. The next day, both birds were still out on their adventure and it continued into the night. Weeks later, there was still no sign of the pigeons. Frances was off seeing the world and wanted to see more.

I won't say that was the defining moment of my childhood but, looking back, it certainly gave me a few ideas. I grew up in a smart working-class home, one where education was viewed as a rare chance to see things beyond my own front door. Higher education, in turn, was the biggest prize – an opportunity to learn and forge a career that would fulfil me and/or do a degree that was both entirely unwanted and unneeded by the labour market.* But I had no sense this was a guarantee. Neither of my parents had gone to university, and I knew no one with a disability who had ever attended. I barely knew anyone with a disability full stop. I filled out my UCAS form with a mix of excitement and doubt, flicking through brochures of places and people that seemed another world away. In the end, I spent over a decade of my life at university. A BA in Political Science at the University of Nottingham turned into an MA, and eventually a PhD. I liked it so much I stayed around to teach. I was once invited on to *Christmas University Challenge* and

* Reader, I did a Political Philosophy PhD.

I only like to mention it twenty times a year. My wings flew further than I could ever have imagined.

Everyone should get the chance to fly. And yet we know that disabled young people who want to go into further education can struggle to access university: from the lack of joined-up disability services, the inaccessibility of lectures and seminars, to being denied adjustments. For disabled students, getting to university takes far more than passing our A levels.

A degree in admin

One thing I realized very quickly at university was that the smallest things made me happy. If the lecture halls included a space at the end of the row that I could slot my wheelchair in. When the student union bar had a stair-lift to enable me to get to the terrace on a warm day. That my graduation gown was made for wheelchair users so the extra length wouldn't get stuck in the wheels. It is not that I had low standards but that I guess I had never taken anything for granted. As a disabled person, I knew the odds of my getting to experience university at all were slim. I was grateful to even be there.

Research suggests that many other disabled young people are missing out. Only around 13 per cent of university students report at least one disability, according to the Office for Students (OfS),[1] compared to the around 18 per cent of the working-age population who are disabled. Of course, not every young person with a disability will want to go into higher education but evidence suggests that being disabled means you might not get the chance. Disabled people are considerably less likely to hold a degree than the general public; only 23 per cent of disabled people aged twenty-one to sixty-four years in the UK have a degree as their highest qualification compared with 40 per cent of people without a disability.[2] Even if we make it to university, we typically face ongoing inequality once we're there. Disabled students are less likely to continue their course, graduate with a good degree, and progress on to a highly skilled job or further study than our non-disabled peers.[3]

It's not hard to see why. Heading off to university and becoming independent for the first time can feel overwhelming for anyone but it can be even more daunting if you have a disability or health condition. If you've chosen a campus away from home, it may mean leaving behind your support network of nearby parents or friends who know you well. It can also mean losing the disability services you had throughout your teens, be it social care or medical teams, and finding yourself having to navigate a whole new adult system in another postcode.

At school, I had an assistant to help me get around and do practical tasks. At university, there was no similar single role and I had no idea what the equivalent was. How could I do my seminar reading if I couldn't reach the library shelves from my wheelchair? What did I do about notes if I wasn't well enough to get to a lecture? I couldn't afford to buy a laptop but the campus PCs weren't accessible so how could I write my essays? It turned out there was support for all of this, but confusingly, they all came from different avenues: some the local council, others central government, and many the university itself. Trying to access disability support at university felt like I was on a Freshers' Week tour but the map was in code. And I had been drinking.

Amelia McLoughlan, Disabled Students UK network director, who herself has cerebral palsy, says this is a common feeling. 'It's clear that the university experience is not designed with disabled or chronically ill students in mind. They can face multiple barriers, from physically inaccessible buildings, lecture materials that aren't in accessible formats, stigma from staff, to huge administrative burdens. There is support available but it can be patchy and varies across different institutions. Disabled students have to navigate what's often a bureaucratic system in order to get support. They must disclose their disability to their university, provide medical evidence, which is often hard to do, and then encounter what's typically lengthy delays in actually getting that support put in place. It all means there often needs to be a sheer Herculean effort by the individual disabled student just to get the support they need. For many, that's simply too much. Navigating this system while successfully completing your degree work can be exhausting, and often comes at a cost to a student's health. They're at a disadvantage to their peers from day one of their course.'

The stats back this up. Research shows many disabled freshers are not even aware of the support that is available to them; a study by the Department for Education showed that just 40 per cent of disabled students knew about Disabled Students' Allowance – the UK government scheme to pay for the extra costs of disability at university – before starting their course.[4] Not receiving help soon enough can have severe consequences for disabled young people. A report by the OfS in 2019 found students with disabilities were having to repeat a year of their degrees due to lack of support, and in some cases had to drop out entirely.[5] The research found that instead of informing eligible students of the help available, universities are too often relying on individuals to disclose their disability and to start and lead the process of being given adjustments themselves.

Nikki Fox, BBC disability news correspondent, who has muscular dystrophy and dyslexia, can identify with this. 'From day one of my music degree I asked to park on a grass verge right in front of my student digs, rather than in the car park, a five-minute walk away on top of a windy hill, but they said no. I couldn't understand. I was a different person at eighteen. Unsure of myself, I was a hot mess – I should've put my foot down and said, "Tough shit, you need to make me a disabled bay outside my flat." But I didn't and that walk to the car park meant I often didn't get to go to my classes because I was just too tired and I knew I'd fall over. I got blown clean off my feet once.

'I struggled to make friends. I had a few boyfriends, realized musicians weren't for me, way too into themselves. I barely went to class. The campus was just too big. I'd often get so close to my next lesson but I'd have walked for such a long time I'd just run out of steam towards the end – my right leg would give way. I'd just have to slowly place myself on the corridor floor, back against a wall, styling that shit out, waiting for a friendly face to ask if they'd mind helping me stand back up again after a ten-minute rest. I'd sit for hours sometimes.

'In the end I told my mum I was pretty sure I was going to fail, and I wasn't going to do that to my parents who had spent money on me they didn't have, in order for me to study. So my mum said, "Come home." She called our local uni and enquired about their music course and I deferred and went there, back into year two. Turns out, when you're five minutes from home and not struggling to walk, wash, cook, clean, make friends, have a life, you can actually study and not do too badly. If I had to do it again, I would most definitely insist on a parking space outside my flat, get funding for a PA. And maybe I'd have started using a mobility scooter a bit sooner. Looking back, I just wanted to please everyone. I still do a bit but not to the detriment of my life and my [health].'

Pippa Stacey, an author and charity consultant, developed ME during her undergraduate degree and knows first-hand the impact health can have on a student's university experience. 'As a non-disabled student I was able to make the most of uni – going out every day, taking part in all the clubs and societies I wanted to, and still really invest time and energy into my studies and my friendships. As a disabled student, every single element of my waking life had to be so carefully moderated while I had to spend my limited energy dealing with the administrative side of accessing support and securing adjustments rather than on my studies or my student life. There would be afternoons that I could have spent working, but instead I'd have to follow up emails with support staff, or deal with literally hundreds of expense receipts, or write apologies for absences and arrange catch-up work. I call it the "diluted" student experience: unlike their non-disabled mates, disabled students have to use their valuable time and energy dealing with barriers, rather than on their studies. When somebody is in that situation, it can feel as though you've lost all the fun bits of the student experience and you're just dealing with the dregs instead – while being surrounded by others your age who seem to be having the best time and living their best life.'

When Stacey asked for adjustments from her university to make this easier, she hit a brick wall. 'I wasn't well enough to attend contact hours, but knew that by conserving energy by staying at home, I could keep on top of things. I asked for my lectures to be recorded so I could study from home, and was told by disability services that this wasn't possible . . . and that if I couldn't physically attend lectures, I should consider taking a year out instead.'

It doesn't have to be this way. With the right support in place, disabled students not only survive higher education – we thrive. After struggling at school, journalist Lucy Webster 'absolutely loved' university. 'I made some brilliant friends in first year who are still my best mates. I loved the course – Politics and International Relations – and societies, coffees between lectures and going to the library only to end up having fun instead of working. We spent an amazing amount of time in the campus pub eating cheesy chips. Disability services ensured I had an accessible room in halls for all three years of my degree, making life very easy as I never had to get transport to lectures. They adapted the room a bit for me, such as changing the light switches to pull cords, and ensured my PAs were given rooms in my flat. They provided staggered deadlines for me; I'm a slow typer and can only do so much per day, so spreading out the work was great. I could also email the library a list of books I needed and they'd have them ready for me to pick up. The Student Union even gave my PAs free tickets for all their events. What made a huge difference, though, was the number of wheelchair users at Warwick – I never felt out of place, and no one really batted an eyelid.'

For many disabled students, university is the first time we are in an environment where there are other disabled people. It can be a revelatory experience. I remember going to an introductory dinner with disabled freshers before the semester started and feeling the strangeness of seeing people my age who looked like me. Coming from a small town, I was used to being the only disabled teenager in the room. Suddenly, we were everywhere. Although disabled young people are still less likely to go to university than others, the number of disabled students is now higher than ever. More than one in every eight students studying in England in 2019 declared at least one disability,[6] while the real number will be even higher as studies show some disabled and chronically ill students are worried about disclosing their condition.[7]

Despite the problems that remain in provision of disability support, higher education is in many ways better equipped than ever to help students with disabilities and health conditions. Mental health services, for example, are becoming much more standard in universities. Natasha Devon MBE, who works in mental health with young people in schools and universities, and who has anxiety herself, has seen significant progress over the last decade. 'As a society, we are light-years ahead of where we were when I went to university in the late 1990s in terms of our understanding of and ability to speak about mental health. Some universities pay the issue lip service at best. But others are super-attentive and proactive. I've just worked with a fairly new campus that actually designed the entire place with student wellbeing at the centre. There are all of these green spaces and quiet zones students have access to, there's counsellors on-campus and all of their permanent staff are trained in Mental Health First Aid. Many universities now offer peer support through student unions and societies, which can be incredibly powerful. I'm a trustee of the charity Student Minds, which has a charter universities can sign up to and which gives them standards of good practice, and also gives students an idea of what provision they have a right to and should expect from their university.'

After her own difficulties at university, Pippa Stacey went on to write *University and Chronic Illness: A Survival Guide*, and recommends several steps for disabled students looking for help: 'Disabled Students' Allowance is a UK-wide scheme for disabled students. You can apply for an allowance online before or during your degree, and if you meet the criteria you'll go on to book a Needs Assessment. If you qualify, the allowance can help fund specialist equipment, one-to-one support, general study expenses, and transport costs. Many universities also offer internal disability services, where an adviser can help you to create a personalized learning plan and support you with any issues that arise. Some universities also offer scholarships, grants and bursaries for disabled students – these will be listed on the finance pages of university websites. Many also have disabled students' groups or societies, and there are an increasing number of small charities and grassroots organizations on social media where students can connect and share their experiences – RAiSE[8] and Disabled Students

UK[9] offer thriving online communities as well as support and information.'

You do not have to figure all this out at once. Trying to get around campus without an assistant during my PhD, I once lost a shoe because I tried to open a door with my foot. (They did not remove my degree at this point.) But I got there, slowly. I applied for funding from the university for a library browser to help get my books, and I was given a note taker for the times I had to miss lectures because of illness. To help with spells of not being well enough to study, I did my MA part-time and took a six-month extension for my PhD. Above anything, I learned there was nothing wrong in needing extra help, and that when I got it, I had an equal shot to everyone else. An equal shot that I deserved.

As this chapter has shown, there are still hurdles facing students with disabilities and health conditions: from the need for more easily accessed adjustments from university disability services to better communication of what funding is available. But we have also seen that with suitable support, and if it is right for our health, young disabled women increasingly can realize their ambitions in higher education – and know there need be no limit to them.

When I was eighteen, I had no idea what the years post-school would be like or how disability would impact me.

You might not either. That's fine. I have come from the future with a secret. Everything will be OK. Even when it doesn't feel like it. *Especially* when it doesn't feel like it. I won't pretend that hurdles won't ever get in the way or that they are always going to be easy to jump but I will say that there is power in taking the routes around the side (and that you will figure them out in your own time). You have more potential inside you than the world can dream of. The next question is, what do you want to do with it?

Careers

'It got to the stage I had applied for over a hundred jobs and I didn't hear anything back. I couldn't understand why. So, I did an experiment and removed any mention of my condition and I was offered an interview and got a job straight away.'
— Shani Dhanda

My career in journalism very much started from the ground up. I don't just mean that in a figurative way. I mean my career literally began with me lying on the ground. In my mid-twenties, and in the final stages of my PhD, I belatedly started thinking about what career I might do. Since the age of seven, I had wanted to be a writer; childhood daydreams scribbled on notepads and an old typewriter. As I entered adulthood, I was none the wiser about how to make it actually happen. Yes, the British media felt like a closed shop, but more than that, as a disabled young person, *any* career felt out of reach. I didn't have the energy to get up early, so how could I do a traditional nine to five? If an employer was based in an older or small building, how could I get in the office with my wheelchair or even reach the desk? My disability meant

I couldn't drive, and much public transport is inaccessible, so how would I get to work?

Unsure and unprepared, I decided to do the only rational thing: apply for an incredibly competitive work experience position in a widely inaccessible city. A bit of googling showed me the *Guardian* newspaper was launching a week's internship in its London offices specifically for disabled applicants; a 'positive action scheme' to help make the workplace less discriminatory. A written application and an in-person interview later, I was offered one of the two spots for the summer. I was elated. The only sticking point: I had nowhere to stay. Based in Nottingham, I had no long-lost relative with a house in Islington and didn't have the strength for a four-hour daily commute. A few friends from university rented flats across the capital but my disability meant they were a no-go; I physically couldn't crash on the sofa or even get up the stairs – with no lift – to get inside. Instead, I stayed in the cheapest hotel I could find. 'Cheapest' in central London meant £500 for five days; money I took from my student loan on the gamble the internship would somehow lead to paid work. That money bought me basic access: a bath I could wash my hair in, and a lift to the breakfast buffet for hash browns. Unfortunately, the bed in the hotel was too high for me to reach from my wheelchair. Housekeeping kindly gave me a substitute – a long cot usually provided for wayward children. For the week, I slept on the floor.

I don't think I'd have a career now if I hadn't taken that risk. In the grand scheme of things, a few uncomfortable nights' sleep was a small inconvenience but it was also an early lesson in the extra hurdles disabled women face in the workplace. As this chapter will show, women with disabilities and health conditions today are making waves across multiple industries – but there are still obstacles to get there. We are routinely paid less than our non-disabled colleagues, can face bullying and harassment, are denied access requirements, and are even less likely to be hired in the first place. Forget a glass ceiling. Too often, this one has a flight of stairs up to it and a sign that says: 'Lift Out of Order'.

Always the work experience girl, never the boss

'How long have you been like *that*?' Sitting in a BBC television green room, the politician opposite gestured to my wheelchair with his eyes. Like many with a visible disability, I'd been in this position before. Intrusive questions from complete strangers is a bizarrely common occurrence for disabled people. It typically revolves around being quizzed on personal medical history, often when you're least expecting it – akin to being asked your favourite sexual position by the postman. It is not only deeply embarrassing – it reflects both a judgement and an entitlement: a disabled person's body is an oddity and public property. In a way, this latest intrusion felt worse because I was at work. This was a safe place. I was Professional Frances here! Dignified! Intelligent! It turns out it is never enough. There is no tailoring of a jacket that can protect a disabled woman from probing questions, no title on an email sign-off that can guarantee respect from every non-disabled person. 'How long have you been like *that*?' he asked. 'Incredible?' I replied, and then paused, deliberately dripping out the words. 'I've been like that for a number of years. How long have you been a bigoted shit fossil?' Of course, I didn't. I mumbled something about being born with a disability as I stared awkwardly out of the window. 'Poor you,' he said, before returning to his newspaper.

What I experienced that afternoon in the green room was a small window into the micro-aggressions disabled people face in the workplace every day. People from ethnic minority backgrounds and women have long reported experiencing micro-aggressions about their race or sex (defined as an indirect or subtle discriminatory comment or behaviour). The disability equivalent rarely gets discussed but disabled employees are just as privy to these sort of underhand – sometimes unintentional – behaviours at work.* Think of a visually impaired manager being told that she 'looks like the work experience girl' or a wheelchair user in a meeting having every question directed to her non-disabled colleague. The thing with small, repeated incidents is that eventually they add up to feel heavy. It becomes exhausting to carry that weight around, as if it

---

* Of course, that also means that disabled female colleagues and disabled women of colour can experience micro-aggressions on multiple identity fronts.

were a ton of concrete strapped to your career that you must drag to the office daily.

Jenny Sealey OBE, who is Deaf, is joint CEO and artistic director of Graeae, the UK's flagship disability-led theatre company, and co-directed the 2012 London Paralympic opening ceremony, has experienced micro-aggressions throughout her long career. 'In my early jobs in theatre, I had very little access to support as I didn't know what access I could get. I'd do workshops with young people with no interpreter. I'm a brilliant lip-reader, but dealing with regional accents and mumbles was a struggle. I had to play catch-up and make sense of what I did manage to get, but it was nerve-racking.

'When I became a director, things improved in some ways – I got access to interpreters – but I felt the micro-aggression of the white non-disabled men who often dominated the room. In the early days of my directing career, if I arrived at meetings with two male interpreters it was perceived by men that they were doing my job and they would only address my signers. If I arrived with women interpreters, it was perceived by men that they were there to care for me and the tone would be kindly and patronizing. I learned to choose very carefully which interpreters I booked for which meetings.

'As my career has progressed, I'm mindful of how my physically impaired employees – especially women directors – take a discriminatory bashing. There seems to be an air of amazement that they are even a director! I have seen people looking over the head of a wheelchair-user director waiting for the "real" director to come in. The big barrier facing us is always the attitudinal barrier.'

At times, this ableist discrimination manifests as outright abuse. Research by the Chartered Institute of Personnel and Development shows disabled people are more than twice as likely to report experiencing bullying or harassment in the workplace than others, with 37 per cent of disabled workers being a victim of such treatment, compared to 18 per cent of non-disabled employees.[1] A separate study by Cardiff University highlighted that the type of disability an individual has can significantly affect their likelihood of experiencing bullying at work. For example, 21 per cent of those with learning disabilities experienced violence at work compared to 10 per cent of disabled workers overall and 5 per cent of those without a disability.[2] For women, this harassment can take specific, ugly forms. Research by the Trades Union Congress (TUC) in 2021 found around seven in ten (68 per cent) disabled women surveyed about sexual harassment say they have been sexually harassed at work,[3] compared to 52 per cent of women in general.[4] The threat is even worse when you're just starting out in your career. Younger disabled women aged eighteen to thirty-four are more likely to have experienced sexual harassment, with almost eight out of ten (78 per cent) reporting being harassed in the workplace. The survey also showed the serious impact this can have; over a third (34 per cent) reported that their most recent experience of sexual harassment negatively affected their mental health, while a shocking one in eight disabled women impacted said they left their jobs because of it.[5]

Rachel Charlton-Dailey, who has multiple chronic conditions including the autoimmune disorder lupus and endometriosis, and is neurodivergent, now works as a journalist but began her work life at a nursery. Her bosses treated her differently to the non-disabled members of staff to the extent she was 'bullied out' of her job. 'The nursery was open from 7 a.m. to 7 p.m., but due to my medication and how much I struggled to sleep with the pain, I couldn't handle early mornings. My managers refused to allow me to only work later shifts and often put me on early shifts straight after I'd had late shifts. If I complained I was treated like I was lazy. When I said that the workload was too much and asked to go part-time, they refused and instead made me "supply staff". It meant I didn't get fixed hours – some weeks I'd have very few hours and others I'd be doing almost forty.

'My deputy manager was especially bullying. Her and a few of the members of staff would openly tease that I wasn't very strong and would trip and stumble a lot, sometimes in front of older children so they thought it was funny to laugh at me too. When I had to take days off, I was treated like I was faking it. Because of how badly I was being treated, I ignored symptoms of my heath deteriorating. I ended up collapsing when I'd been left alone in a room with twelve children. I was so scared to go home when I was ill, for fear of being fired, that I had passed out. I later found out I'd suffered a mini stroke. When I told my boss her response was, "Oh, so you'll be missing more work." It was the most toxic environment I've ever been in.'

There are multiple factors that may explain why colleagues and bosses feel they can freely discriminate against women with disabilities and health conditions, but one is surely that there are often still too few disabled people in the room. While the last fifty years have seen enormous progress from the days of disabled people being segregated from society and excluded from the workplace, we are still 'the odd ones out' in most professions. As a rare disabled woman working in the media, I'm still often The Only Disabled in the Room, especially in a senior position. But journalism is far from the only industry to have a disability problem. A minute 0.5 per cent of teachers self-report as having disabilities in the UK, compared with an estimated 16 per cent of working-age adults in the general population.[6] Only around 2 per cent of the healthcare workforce in NHS England disclose a disability or long-term health condition, although – just as with all self-reported figures – it's estimated there will be more doctors and nurses out there who have not publicly reported their disability.[7]

Meanwhile, there are no executives or senior managers who have disclosed a disability at any of the FTSE 100 companies, as of 2021,[8] while on average only 3.2 per cent of their employees have disabilities. This is the case across the board in business. The proportion of employers who say their organization employs any disabled staff at all was just 33 per cent in 2020.[9]

This inequality only ramps up once you get to senior positions in the workplace. In most organizations, minorities like disabled women are still concentrated at the bottom and get increasingly rarer the further up the ladder we look. Even companies who appear to have a track record of 'diversity' are often less progressive about hiring women with disabilities to senior and leadership roles. Evidence shows that disabled people are generally less likely to be employed as managers, directors or senior officials, or to be employed in professional occupations full stop. Just over one-quarter (25.7 per cent) of employed disabled people hold these positions in the UK, in comparison with just under one-third (32.3 per cent) of employed non-disabled people, according to the ONS.[10] Instead, people with disabilities and long-term health conditions are more likely to be in lower-skilled, part-[11] or low-paid work;[12] shockingly, nearly three-quarters (72 per cent) of disabled workers earn less than the median wage of £15 an hour, according to analysis of official statistics published by the TUC in 2022.[13] At the same time, disabled people are also more likely to be on zero-hours contracts[14] – even more so if you're a woman of colour.[15] Don't let anyone ever tell you there is some sort of shame in these jobs – putting a shift in as a cleaner, let alone when you're in chronic pain, is hard, valuable work – but structural inequality means it is women with disabilities who are more likely to do them, often with little chance of ever having senior and secure roles.

If you're disabled, finding a job at all can be a feat. The disability employment gap is staggering: only around half (52.2 per cent) of disabled people are in paid work in the UK, compared to four in five (80.9 per cent) non-disabled people. Even fewer young people with disabilities are in the labour force. According to the ONS, the employment rate among disabled 18–24-year-olds was 46.4 per cent in 2019, versus 71 per cent among non-disabled people of the same age.

There are multiple reasons for this employment gap, Joanna Owen, a solicitor who has worked for the Equality and Human Rights Commission (EHRC), and is tetraplegic from a spinal cord injury, explains: 'It can go back all the way to childhood where disabled students don't always get the same opportunities to do well at school or university. For example, a child with a visual impairment may want a career in IT but if they don't get the right computer software at school, they won't be able to follow everything in class to get the right qualifications. Unsurprisingly, this puts us at a disadvantage when we start looking for work opportunities. Companies and employers are also not yet flexible enough to make some of the adjustments that people with disabilities and health conditions need. For example, adaptive technology or different work patterns to accommodate longer breaks. So disabled people who are otherwise really qualified for these jobs just might not be able to take them.

'The employment gap can also be because employers make assumptions about disabled job applicants without giving us a chance to prove our abilities, so there's a discriminatory situation where some employers are less likely to hire someone if they're disabled or even give them an interview. In some cases, this can be unlawful.

'Women are likely to be more affected by the disability employment gap. Women have traditionally been less likely than men to apply for jobs they don't feel qualified for (even when they are) or push themselves forward for promotions in the workplace, and having a disability as well may compound that. Women – including disabled ones – also are far more likely than men to have caring responsibilities for children, their parents or partners, and that affects our career chances too.

'A small minority of disabled and chronically ill people can't work because of their health, which will account for a tiny aspect of the employment gap. But it's a myth that disabled people can't contribute to the workplace, especially with the right support. There are fantastic disabled candidates out there who are just as able and talented as their non-disabled counterparts but just aren't getting the same opportunities.'

Shani Dhanda – who was born with brittle bones – is now an award-winning disability specialist and entrepreneur. But when she left school at sixteen, she struggled to be taken seriously by employers. 'I thought the best thing to do would be to include the fact I had a condition but needed no adjustments in my covering letter. I thought it would help remove any awkwardness at the interview because I have short stature and people are super-awkward or nervous around me. It got to the stage I had applied for over a hundred jobs and I didn't hear anything back. I couldn't understand why.

'So, I did an experiment and removed any mention of my condition and I was offered an interview and got a job straight away. I had to learn a harsh life lesson at sixteen that people were going to judge my ability on the fact I have a condition. It left me feeling hopeless and I was worried about my future, because if I struggled to get a part-time job how was I going to survive in life? It gave me the mindset for my career: I can't rely on other people to give me opportunities, I needed to create my own.'

This discrimination in hiring practices is all too common. One in five (22 per cent) business leaders in the UK would be unlikely to hire someone with a known disability, according to research by recruitment firm PageGroup in 2021.[16] The main reasons for this are a lack of internal support systems and fears over the costs of modifying equipment to accommodate disabled employees, as well as a perception that disabled people may lack the right skills. This flagrant bias means talented disabled candidates like Dhanda have to send out 60 per cent more CVs than non-disabled people on average before they find a job.[17] It's no wonder that one study found 77 per cent of disabled applicants are fearful of disclosing their disability to prospective employers.[18] Being a disabled jobseeker is a hell of a lot of work.

On top of the biased attitudes of prospective employers, disabled workers have to contend with practicalities too. Research by Samsung in 2022[19] found disabled people still face a range of access problems at work: from a lack of quiet areas in the office (33 per cent); stairs or lack of space (32 per cent); toilet access (30 per cent); and even getting into the office building (29 per cent). At the same time, there's often significant gaps in support outside the workplace, such as disability benefits and social care, that affect how people with disabilities and health conditions can get by day-to-day. This naturally has a knock-on effect on how easy it is for us to build a career. If you can't get your wheelchair on to the Tube, the London commute can be impossible. Without social care funding for a personal assistant, there's no one to help you get dressed for the office in the morning.*

Every job interview or opportunity I've ever had has hung on the question of whether my body will be accommodated. Will there be an accessible toilet nearby or will I have to withhold liquids for the day? If I stay overnight, will I have access to an adapted bath or will I have to meet the interviewer with greasy hair? Will the train to get to the meeting have an available wheelchair space, and if not, will the next one that does come in time? As a disabled woman, how qualified I am for a job has always come second to whether there's a lift to get to the interview.

This cocktail of social attitudes and structural inequality doesn't just mean it's hard to get a job if you're disabled. It also makes it harder to stay in work, and get back into work if you fall out of it. Figures from the ONS show disabled workers in the UK move out of work at nearly twice the rate (8.8 per cent) of non-disabled workers (4.9 per cent), while unemployed disabled people move into work at nearly one-third of the rate (11.0 per cent) of non-disabled people (26.9 per cent).[20] Young people are all too aware of this. Research by the disability charity Leonard Cheshire in

---

* Research shows wider access has a quantifiable impact on our career opportunities. One study found a disabled person is four times more likely to be in work if their accessible housing needs are met: https://thiis.co.uk/habinteg-finds-wheelchair-users-subjected-to-decades-long-wait-for-new-accessible-housing

2021[21] found less than half (49 per cent) of young disabled people think they would find another job if they became unemployed.

The result isn't simply that disabled women have to face lower incomes and insecurity during our working lives, but afterwards too. Research by the pension company Scottish Widows in 2023[22] found more than half (51 per cent) of disabled people struggle to save enough for retirement throughout their careers, with disabled workers almost twice as likely to be priced out of an adequate retirement as non-disabled workers (51 per cent versus 28 per cent).

I've listed a lot of statistics there and not just to prove I did in fact pass GCSE maths. Data about employment is useful to give an accurate picture of what's going on in the world. But they also tell us something else: it is not your fault. One of the most crucial survival skills for disabled women in a non-disabled space is to understand how institutional ableism works. When you know that statistically an employer is less likely to hire you if you're disabled, you know you probably didn't screw up that interview like you told yourself you did when you read the rejection email. When you are sending out fifty CVs and hearing nothing back, you can see it in the context of how many more job applications disabled candidates have to make on average than our non-disabled competitors. This isn't to say we are helpless. On the contrary, knowing the factors that affect our lives gives us power. It stops us wasting our time beating ourselves up over things that we are not to blame for. It lets us know the structural inequality at play in the workplace and helps us put our energy towards challenging it. As Alice Wong, an activist, editor and writer, who uses a wheelchair and a tracheostomy, puts it to me: 'Being overlooked, excluded or underestimated is commonplace to me. It's shitty but it forces me to fight for myself and others, know what I want and why I want it, celebrate my excellence and know my value when others don't.'

Jane Hatton, who has a spinal condition, runs the social enterprise Evenbreak, which helps disabled people into new or better work, and like Wong, encourages women with disabilities and health conditions receiving job rejections to recognize their own value – or as she says, to see themselves as 'premium candidates'. 'We know that employers and recruiters can have negative views of disabled people. They've been conditioned by the perception that we are somehow "less" than non-disabled people, and worry that we might not be productive, have loads of time off sick, or cost a fortune in adjustments. Even worse is that sometimes we also buy into that narrative. But we have the same diverse range of skills and talents as the rest of the population, and often added determination and problem-solving skills.'

Hatton suggests four actions for anyone with a health condition struggling to find a job. 'Firstly, we need to focus our mind on all of the strengths and benefits we bring to a role so that we can apply with confidence, knowing we would be a huge asset to the employer. Secondly, we need to make sure the recruiter knows about this too. Be specific about those qualities that make you a premium candidate, and don't be shy about promoting these to the recruiter. Thirdly, there are specialist job boards where enlightened employers are proactively looking to attract disabled candidates, so it's worth searching those out. Finally, don't be afraid to ask for what you need if the recruitment processes are inaccessible to you. And ask in a positive, not apologetic, way. Less "I'm really sorry, I'm going to need . . ." and more "I'll be able to perform at my best if I have . . ." If the employer doesn't offer you the adjustments you need for the recruitment process, you know that this is not the place for you. We deserve employers who value us.'

Because you're worth it

If there's one – often tricky – way to value ourselves in the workplace, it's negotiating a pay rise. It's a well-known fact that women earn less than men.[23] The true gender pay gap is hard to get an exact figure on, but, when comparing equally qualified people doing the same job, most estimates by labour economists and data analysis put it at somewhere between 10 per cent and 20 per cent.[24] While the gender pay gap has thankfully been given more attention in recent years, we talk much less about the disability pay gap – that is, the difference between how much disabled workers and their non-disabled colleagues earn – and even less so about how sex and disability combine uniquely to hit disabled women's bank balances. It's common now for brands and companies – particularly those aimed at a female audience – to get behind Equal Pay Day, monetizing inequality with an Instagram hashtag. But I can't remember ever seeing a disabled woman used in these campaigns, or the role of physical or mental health conditions mentioned as an issue we should be tackling. Equal-pay initiatives are in many ways 'equal pay for non-disabled women'.

The lack of attention given to disability in discussion of the gender pay gap is particularly frustrating considering disabled women are disproportionately affected by it. Non-disabled employees in the UK earn on average £1.90 an hour more than disabled employees – or a sixth of total pay – according to research by the TUC in 2023.[25] That's the equivalent of disabled workers losing out on £3,460 a year based on a 35-hour week – or several months' rent. Disabled women face an even bigger pay gap compared specifically to men. Non-disabled men are paid on average £3.50 an hour – or around £6,370 a year – more than disabled women.[26] That means that while the average woman faces a 10–20 per cent pay gap to men, disabled women are losing a colossal 30 per cent.[27]

It's illegal to pay a disabled person less for doing a job of equal value to a non-disabled person – instead, the disability pay gap is caused by more sneaky, indirect factors. Disabled people and women are more likely to need to work part-time, which can see them be discriminated against when it comes to climbing up the pay scales, with higher-level jobs often not available on part-time hours. Meanwhile, lower-paid jobs, such as cleaning and caring, are mainly done by women (and often black and migrant women), while higher-paid jobs are – surprise, surprise – traditionally seen as male. On top of this, disabled workers can miss out on the chance for promotion if employers deny them the simple adjustments they need to do their job, such as assistive technology or flexible hours. Put together, it all means disabled women are often stuck on the lowest rungs of the pay ladder.

Dr Amy Kavanagh, who is blind, works as a freelance disability consultant, and has repeatedly experienced pay discrimination – and even been asked to work for nothing. 'I'm constantly asked to do work for free. Sometimes it's by charities, often by private companies. Early on in my career, I took some of these jobs, believing their line that it would help me with "exposure". Eventually, I realized how much I was giving away. Recently, I was asked to speak on a panel about accessibility at an international online conference. This event was primarily for media companies, including some streaming giants, so a multi-billion-dollar industry. After delaying and dithering for four weeks, making me hold time in my diary, constantly chasing with emails, they told me not only that they wouldn't agree to my fee but that they wouldn't pay me at all for my time on the panel. I was one of the few disabled people scheduled to speak at the entire event, the rest of the speakers were corporate execs doing it as part of a full-time paid role. Yet they didn't want to pay the disabled person. It was grossly insulting.

'It's like there's an assumption that disabled people will be grateful for any work. It's the ableism of a society that thinks I'm sat in the dark being a sad blind person just waiting for some attention and that I'll be overjoyed to give up hours of time for free. And that I don't have a mortgage or a family or a social life like other people that I need to pay for. Luckily I have found projects and businesses willing to recognize my value and expertise and reflect that through my pay, but I'm shocked at how often I'm still asked to do work for free.'

Being asked to work for nothing would be galling for anyone, but even more so when you need more cash than most. Research by Scope in 2023[28] found that disabled households with at least one disabled adult or child face extra costs of £975 a month on average – the equivalent to 63 per cent of our income, after housing costs. Let's call it the 'disability tax': on top of paying utility bills, food, rent and socializing like everyone else, disabled people have to stretch our income to buy anything from accessible transport, regular physio, to disability equipment.

Against this backdrop, being able to negotiate our pay is a particularly useful skill for disabled women. However, research consistently suggests women are less likely to ask for a raise. One study[29] carried out by Good Money Week, a campaign which shines a light on ethical finance, in 2021 found 41 per cent of men had talked about a salary rise with their manager in the last six months, whereas just a third of women had. Women notably had negative feelings about approaching the subject: nearly a third of women feel 'awkward' about asking for more money but just a fifth of men feel uncomfortable.[30] It's hardly a surprise many women feel this way. From when we are little girls, we are praised for being 'polite' and scolded for seeming 'bossy'. And yet the problem is not simply that women are not speaking up – research shows that even when women do ask for a pay rise they are less likely to get one than men, and judged more harshly for asking. A YouGov survey in 2022[31] found one in five women who ask for a pay rise are successful in receiving one compared with just under a third of men. Even requesting a raise can be detrimental if you're female. Research at Harvard University found women who do lobby for either a raise or a higher starting salary are more likely than men to be perceived as greedy, demanding or just not very nice.[32] What's 'assertive' for a man is 'pushy' for a woman.

Predictably, women with disabilities can find it even harder to get on at work. Research by Samsung in 2022[33] – which surveyed both disabled women and men – found many worry their health will impact their chances of moving up the career ladder; over half of people with disabilities (45 per cent) surveyed have actually tried to conceal their condition from work colleagues due to the fear of stalling their professional progression or landing a promotion. As is so often the case, there is little research specifically about what disabled women are experiencing at work, but anecdotally, women with health conditions face the double hit of social attitudes towards disability and gender that judge them as less likely to be 'promotion material'. 'There is an erroneous assumption that disabled people are so grateful to actually have a job, that we are not interested in fair pay or career progression,' says Jane Hatton. 'But we should enjoy the same rights and respect at work as everyone else . . . It's a case of knowing your value and making sure others know it too. We aren't raised to be boastful, and that's particularly true as disabled women. Well, as the saying goes, "Shy girls get nowt!", so we need to demonstrate we have the same diverse range of aspirations and ambitions as everyone else. And the same rights to opportunities to achieve them.'

Rachael Mole, who has Ehlers–Danlos syndrome and the heart condition postural tachycardia syndrome (PoTS), is the founder of Moleworks Solutions, a company that helps increase disability inclusion in the workplace, and she says there are a number of practical steps disabled women can take to negotiate a pay rise with confidence. 'First, it's an emotionally draining situation to be in, so step away for a few beats if you need to so you don't do anything you may later regret (hello, profanity-filled resignation email). The next thing you need to do is your research. What are your colleagues who are in the same job as you earning? Have you taken on any additional tasks and duties you aren't being remunerated for? Has one of your ideas brought value to the organization? How long have you been with the organization? What is the market rate for this job? What is the figure you want to be earning?

'Compile it all in a report, ready to present the business case. If you could walk into another job, with another company, and earn more than you're being paid here, then what is your current company going to do to make sure that doesn't happen? Email your manager to ask for a meeting – paper trails from this point onwards are so important as it will then all be on record. Finally, when a new salary offer is made, thank them, and ask for a few days to consider it. This is expected, and you should never feel pressured to take it right then and there. They are starting negotiations, and if they can't budge on the number then suggest additional non-monetary compensation, like more paid holiday days.'

If you're not disabled yourself but want to be an ally, there are ways you can help your disabled colleagues get fairer pay. For example, consider sharing your salary number with close disabled colleagues.* It can feel awkward to talk about

---

* According to the TUC, one in five workers in Britain have gag clauses in their contract, effectively banning them from talking about pay. Check your contract first!

money – one poll[34] found only one-third of people surveyed said they would discuss their salary with colleagues – but pay transparency is one of the best ways to tackle unequal pay for marginalized employees. If disabled women know how much more their non-disabled colleagues are earning for doing the same role, it gives us added bargaining muscle to negotiate a pay rise. The clichés are sometimes true: knowledge is power.

If you don't ask

When I first started out in my career, I was reluctant to ask for anything. I didn't want to say I couldn't reach the button that controlled the PowerPoint display because I was too low in my wheelchair. I didn't want to admit I needed long sick leave even as I was lying in bed. I think it was a fear of being seen as 'high maintenance' mixed with embarrassment. The embarrassment of being different.

Whether it's in the workplace or outside of it, many of us with disabilities are used to preceding an access request with the word 'sorry'. We often don't even know we're doing it. 'Sorry, do you have an accessible loo?' 'Really sorry but I'll need an extra ticket for my PA.' It is an apology for existing, a 'While I'm in the office, I will need regular access to air containing 21 per cent oxygen. Sorry for being such a pain!'

It is easy to feel self-conscious if your health condition means that you need modifications at work, or to worry that it will be detrimental to your career. Asking for what we need as disabled women can feel intimidating in a world that too often labels us 'difficult' and 'ungrateful' if we push for more. It's not as if these worries are irrational; minorities are all too aware that we may be punished for sticking our heads above the line. That fear can be even stronger at the beginning of your career when you're still trying to prove yourself and your position feels less secure. While everyone else is just thinking about promotions and pay rises, disabled women have to worry about whether our bosses will even give us the adjustments we need to do our job.

Here's the good news: it's your legal right. In the majority of developed nations, campaigning by disabled activists over recent decades means there are now legal protections for disabled workers – including the right to have some modifications in the workplace. In the UK, the Equality Act 2010 gives disabled people the right to what are called 'reasonable adjustments', while the US has similar legislation in the Americans with Disabilities Act (ADA) 1990.

Lib Whitfield, who has endometriosis and bipolar, and runs equality campaigns for the trade union GMB, explains: 'By law, employers are required to make reasonable adjustments for disabled employees and job applicants. Adjustments can be as simple as having a different chair due to a back condition, having text-to-speech software or even just not being able to work certain shift patterns, like nights. What is "reasonable" varies – for example, it can depend on the size and therefore budget of the employer – but it generally means it is simple to make and of low cost. The duty is on the employer to show it would be unreasonable for them to manage to make an adjustment.

'It's best to say what you need at the earliest stage possible. Getting adjustments might begin with a conversation with your line manager or prospective employer. Larger employers may have occupational health teams that they will refer you to and make what we call a "reasonable adjustment passport", a document that lists the adjustments that you need so that any manager you work with from then on will be able to see what's been agreed. It can be more difficult gaining adjustments from very small employers whose finances are limited, or if you're on a zero-hours contract, but remember any worker has this legal right. Because disabilities and needs can change over time, employees should also be given the opportunity to have their adjustments regularly reviewed in a positive way.'

Dr Hannah Barham-Brown, a GP and TEDx speaker on disability in the workplace, has ADHD and uses a wheelchair due to Ehlers–Danlos syndrome and the nervous system condition dysautonomia, and knows first-hand how to advocate for adjustments at work. 'I work what the NHS call Less Than Full Time (LTFT) clinically – so effectively three days a week – because I become exhausted and seize up if I work more than that. In my current GP job, I also do fewer home visits as most houses aren't wheel-chair accessible – so we've prioritized me being the one to do visits to patients in care homes and nursing homes, as they tend to be accessible! I start and end my clinic an hour later, working from 10 to 6, as I know my body takes a while to get going in the mornings. I have a work laptop at home with access to our computer systems, so if my body is having a particularly silly day and getting into the surgery isn't looking likely but my brain is still up for it, I can do a telephone clinic from home. This is great if I have a random dislocation with my EDS.

'These adjustments have all come about informally, gen-erally by sitting down early on with bosses and talking through what might work for us both. I try to keep lines of communication open, so if I find something new that might help, or something that isn't working for me, we can try to find solutions together. It's often very hard for medics to get the adjustments they need, particularly when you're starting out because of the rotating nature of our training, and moving teams and locations frequently. A recent British Medical Association (BMA) report I helped put together found that only 55 per cent of doctors get the reasonable adjustments they need. I passionately believe that health-care is at its best when the diversity of our staff reflects the diversity of our patients. I've had patients tell me they trust me and engage with me because they know I "get it". As such, I wear my queer, neurodivergent, wheelchair-using identity with pride.'

Ruth Golding, a senior leader in a secondary school and co-founder of disabled education network DisabilityEd UK, who has primary lymphoedema in her limbs, shares this attitude in her own profession. 'In the classroom, I teach seated rather than walking around and circulating the class. I have reduced duties or they are adapted, such as doing a detention [where I can sit down] so that my legs get a rest. I have flexibility around start times when needed; for example, I can start later after a parents' evening because my legs swell and become painful. I've also had air conditioning fitted to cool the room to prevent my limbs swelling. These adaptations help me to do my best work but I wasn't always comfortable asking for them. It took me the best part of forty years to truly embrace my disabled identity, and I am better at asking now than I was at the start of my career.

'In the ableist world that disabled people live in we can be crippled with the low self-esteem of not feeling valued. At the same time, people don't always feel comfortable with declaring a disability to their bosses, or think of themselves as disabled, or are just not fully aware of their rights. This all definitely makes it harder to ask for adjustments. But having more disabled teachers benefits the whole school: with over 22 per cent of students being disabled, they deserve to see themselves in the people who teach them. To disabled teachers or those thinking about a career, I'd say don't be afraid to be open about your disability and needs. Most importantly remember you are worth it, you

are not a problem – you are simply asking to not experience discrimination.'

As a former adviser to President Obama, Alice Wong, who
uses a wheelchair and a tracheostomy, is proof that adaptations for disabled staff are possible in the highest-level
jobs – even the White House. After working remotely from
San Francisco, California for several years, Wong received
an email from the White House inviting her to an important event in Washington DC. 'I didn't reply because I live
[on the other side of the country] . . . I use a power chair
and no longer fly because the risks are too great for my
health, even though the FOMO is a real thing. [But the
White House team] followed up with me and mentioned
that they made arrangements for a telepresence robot for
me to operate from my laptop for the event. I never had
the opportunity to use one and this was before live streaming and video conferencing was commonplace. It was one
of the most exciting experiences of my life and much of
it was due to having disabled people in decision-making
positions who are proactive about accessibility. There have
been many events and opportunities I missed [but] this
one was centred on and organized by the community. This
made all the difference.'

Throughout her long career, Wong has learned to
advocate for herself in the workplace, and be unapologetic
about her needs. 'There's little about the way I sound, look
and show up in spaces where I can hide any aspect of my

identities. I am always upfront about my access needs and who I am.'

Despite such vast gains when it comes to access for disabled workers in recent decades, it's clear there's further progress to be made. There is limited research on how many disabled people currently have the modifications at work that they need, but from what we do know, many are still struggling. One survey in 2022 found two in five disabled employees in the UK were not receiving the reasonable adjustments they need from their employer.[35] That's anything from missing out on more control over their work schedule, more patience and understanding from others, clearer communication, to additional time for some tasks. Meanwhile, research by UNISON found that 67 per cent of its disabled members had been turned down for some or all of the adjustments they needed. Even where the employer agreed to provide adjustments, nearly a quarter waited a year or more for them to be put in place.[36] We also know adjustments aren't given equally: data by the ONS in 2023[37] found that – while flexible working had increased since the pandemic – workers on salaries of more than £50,000, people with degrees, Londoners and white people had the highest rates of home or hybrid working and were less likely to be required to go in every day.

Lib Whitfield says there are several steps that disabled workers can take if we come up against resistance from bosses. 'If your employer refuses to make reasonable adjustments, it is important to get this decision and their reasons in writing as they have to show the adjustments would be unreasonable for them to make (either for cost or other reasons). With many employers, you can then raise a grievance or appeal against this decision and ask someone more senior to look at the decision again. If your request is still refused you can consider taking legal action in an employment tribunal for discrimination. Joining a trade union is hugely helpful for this, as they will represent, support and advise you of your rights at every step throughout a process of gaining reasonable adjustments – and sometimes even fund your legal case. It can be stressful trying to manage this on your own, especially when managing a disability as well.'

It took many years for me to feel comfortable asking for adjustments at work. Nowadays, I regularly do: from setting out times of the day I'm out of email contact because I'm resting, asking for my personal assistant's travel expenses to be covered, to taking meetings over the phone or Zoom rather than in-person when it's better for my health. I realized, slowly, that I deserved to be on a level footing with my non-disabled colleagues, and that advocating for myself was a crucial part of having a positive experience at work and looking after my body. I realized I was a valuable part of any team and it was in my *employer's* interests to make our workplace accessible for me. Above all, I understood that access is not some "favour" non-disabled people are kindly bestowing upon us – it's our legal right.

As disabled women, we can spend much of our careers trying to fit in – to be as little 'trouble' as possible to our bosses or to not seem different from our colleagues. But the truth is, the workplace was not built with us in mind. We can shrink ourselves until there is barely anything left and still not fit the structures that were made for non-disabled people. So why not just be you? You were hired because you are valued and have earned your place (probably ten times over). You have no need to justify yourself for however your body works. You are not an inconvenience. You are not demanding either. You are a capable professional who knows the adjustments that will enable you to do your job brilliantly. Advocate for what you need, take it, and watch yourself fly. Rather than fitting in, let's stand out.

There was a moment, somewhere between filing a news investigation and finding Oreo crumbs in my bed, that I realized 'workplace adjustments' don't always come with a sign-off by HR. As life-changing as the sort of adaptations we've been discussing have been for the disabled community, the reality is that many of the modifications that workers with disabilities and health conditions rely on aren't official or even the result of conversations with employers. They are the product of our own ingenuity; a toolkit of piecemeal solutions built up over years and 'right, I can't do it like that, but how about like this' thinking that sees disabled women not only survive in the workplace every day but thrive. That they are often out of sight does not mean they are not happening, or that they are even new; almost a century ago, Frida Kahlo had an adapted easel so she could paint while being horizontal in bed.[38]

Baroness Jane Campbell, who uses a wheelchair and BiPAP to breathe, sits in Parliament as an independent cross-bench member of the House of Lords, but often ends up governing from home. 'As somebody who relies totally on another person to function in terms of moving, eating, drinking, writing, and sometimes speaking when I am running out of puff, I rely on what I call a great deal of human assistance time in my working day. I have a part-time support worker plus a PA, both funded by different schemes, that enables me to carry out all my duties as a parliamentarian. These days I can't move except one finger, so my PAs facilitate pretty much everything, from writing letters, looking up files, preparing me for interviews, making phone calls, and conveying messages when I am too tired to speak. My brain seems to be working OK but my body often says "no" at very inconvenient times! I also have someone to read out my speech in Parliament when I get breathless. I'm currently working to find a computer program that sounds like me and could read my speeches or parliamentary questions.

'During the coronavirus pandemic [lockdowns], Parliament went virtual which means I'm now able to participate in parliamentary work via online [Zoom-style] screens if my health means I'm not able to be there in person. I give speeches in the Lords Chamber or join in select committees all from my own home.'

As a broadcast journalist, Emma Barnett has presented BBC flagship current affairs programmes on both radio and television. What her audience may not know is she lives with endometriosis and is often dealing with pain as she works. 'My toolkit is heat and pills. And occasionally a hot sweet drink. I take drugs, sit down a lot more often, and sometimes take myself to the loo for privacy – to breathe through the pain. When I'm presenting radio I have been known to have a hot-water bottle below the desk when pain is very bad . . . I don't even mention it unless someone asks me about it. I also broadcast with my chair at an angle slightly back too – so the hot-water bottle can balance. I look slightly rude-girl!

'The thing I have grown more confident about is showing how I feel on my face. Colleagues who know me well, before the performance as it were, see the grimace. [I've also grown more confident at] telling colleagues how I feel – that has come with the sad knowledge it ain't getting better. I can still function but I can't spare the energy to pretend off-air that I am OK. Because I need it all for on-air.'

It takes nerve to 'show the grimace'. Most of us have spent at least some of our time trying to fit in at work, shifting and squirming to conform to how other people are, to what other bodies do. I often think there is a pressure to 'pass' as a non-disabled person at times – to head into the workplace and act the same as our colleagues who have very different lives and needs. That pressure is easy to buy into ourselves. I've been chronically ill for seven years now, on top of the disability I was born with, and I still have days where I expect my body to behave as if it were healthy. Where I am genuinely shocked to learn that having severe fatigue means I might get exhausted after a work phone call and need a break. I'm essentially one of those dogs who has her leg amputated only to still jump out of my basket and try and run. It is a sign of how powerful ableist messages can be that we are often conditioned to feel embarrassed by the adaptations we need because of our health when, really, we deserve to feel pride. Disabled women are out there taking the normal rules of the workplace and rejecting them, respecting our value and doing things on our own terms – and in the process, doing *great* things.

Of course, there's a privilege to being able to work in a way that fits with your disability. Many jobs, particularly those with lower pay or limited security, are still inflexible and, with it, tough for many people with health conditions. If you wait tables to pay the bills, you can't exactly do it from the comfort of your bed. But it is in everyone's interests – including employers – to do all we can to help adapt the workplace to be as friendly to disabled workers as possible. When businesses make themselves suitable for employees with disabilities, they're not doing a charitable favour – they're making the smart move to get as much disabled talent through their doors as they can. At the same time, they're generally getting employees who have a special set of transferable skills. If you can only use one arm, it isn't a stereotype to say you're probably a better problem-solver than most. If you've got limited energy, you soon learn how to be efficient to get things done. When more bosses understand that disability is just a different – not lesser – way of living, they may realize that their work-place will improve, not from keeping disabled people out, but actively bringing them in. As Lara Parker, deputy director of BuzzFeed US, who has endometriosis, puts it to me: 'I firmly believe that people living with any sort of chronic illness can be just as productive and crucial to any organization because we naturally know how to multitask and work quickly and efficiently. [After all], we've been doing this in our own lives for years.'

Rest is a full-time job

'What do you want to be when you grow up?' From child-hood, we are conditioned to picture a career as a key part of our lives. Nurse. Firefighter. Space cowboy. When we become adults, this only accelerates. The first thing people ask a stranger at a party is 'What do you do for a living?' I've even followed these rules in this book to a certain extent: right between a person's name and disability, I've men-tioned what they do for work. But what if your health means you're not able to hold down a job, let alone develop a career? This issue has become increasingly relevant in recent years. A record high of 2.6 million people in the UK are out of work because of long-term health conditions as of 2024,[39] with another 3.9 million people in employment but with a health condition that limits the type or amount of work they can do[40] – an increase of 1.5 million since just over a decade ago.[41]

This is not just about people ageing as they near retirement. Many affected are young people at the start of their careers: the number of under-35s out of work because of sickness[42] soared by 44 per cent to more than 560,000 between 2019 and 2023 (which experts put down to worsening mental health and underinvestment in health services). As *The Times* put it in 2024 (with some concern), young women are now more likely to be off work due to illness than because they are working after children.[43]

There is a deep social stigma attached to not being able to have a job. We live in a culture that equates work with identity and self-worth, where busyness is a hallmark of value and rest is often frowned upon. Apps track our productivity, while social media offers us 'life hacks' to always keep striving. Even online feminism has been co-opted by this hyper-capitalist message over the last decade. Be a girl boss! Slay! Hustle! How about we all have a lovely lie-down? This messaging is intense for anyone but it can be all the more difficult if you're dealing with health problems. On top of the same pressures facing the wider public, those of us with disabilities face unique demands from society to 'contribute' – often defined as holding down a paid job – and can experience particularly harsh judgements if we 'fail' to. This manifests culturally in accusations that disabled people who can't work are lazy or 'scroungers' and could surely do more if only they tried harder; ideas that in recent years have made it into popular culture through television,[44] newspapers,[45] and even politicians' speeches.[46] As government minister Laura Trott put it in 2023, disabled people must 'do their duty' and work.[47]

At the same time, this rhetoric can impact disabled people who are employed but work reduced hours. As disabled women, it can feel as if we have to be exceptional in the workplace just to prove we are as adequate as anyone else. It's not enough to simply have a job – there is an obligation to work ever harder and better to 'prove' ourselves in order to counter prejudice that we aren't as driven or capable as others; after all, research shows around one in three (32 per cent) members of the public think that disabled people are not as productive as non-disabled people at least some of the time.[48] It all adds up to mean that, if you're chronically ill or disabled, it can be hard to avoid the pressure to follow the 'normal rules' of work: build a career; be productive; work full-time; don't take breaks. Even if our bodies have other ideas.

When everyone around her seemed to be 'hustling' for 'their best life', the gut condition Crohn's disease meant

Ione Gamble was spending twenty hours a day in bed. Now an author and podcaster looking at feminism, health and culture, Gamble is keenly aware of the pressure to be productive. 'In the second half of the 2010s, at a time when social media was enveloping our lives, we saw a wave of what we might call commercialized feminism – think "girl boss and personal branding" – targeted at women who were just entering adulthood. The message was we should be climbing the career ladder as quickly and as successfully as you can, and that we always have to be "on". These narratives are so often toxic as they require us to constantly be optimizing our existences; to be working on our careers from home, after we've left our day job. They raise the bar of expectation far beyond what is possible for anyone with health issues – leading us to have problems in the workplace as well as in our personal relationships. These narratives are also rooted in individualism; that if you, personally, work hard enough and want it enough, you can do whatever you want. As disabled and chronically ill people know, this is simply untrue.

'I myself absolutely felt the pressure to build a career and constantly be productive. I had to quit my first adult job as I realized the requirements to work in a "normal" office environment were entirely impossible for me to adhere to, and that I had to construct a way for myself to live that was completely non-typical from what most other people do with their time. I still feel the pressure to be productive and to keep the pedal on when it comes to my career, but I have learned to be a lot easier on myself. I think social media encourages so much comparison and competition that even if you aren't spending all day in bed it can feel like you aren't doing enough. But really taking time to think about it, and to take on the tasks you're able to do the best you can, I think it becomes easy to realize that never giving yourself a break is actually harmful, means the work you are doing isn't good, and won't help you in the long run.'

As Gamble says, the push to be endlessly busy isn't just bad for our wellbeing – it's counterproductive. Research consistently shows that overworking doesn't actually make us better at our jobs (and sometimes it even makes us worse). In his book *Rest: Why You Get More Done When You Work Less*, Alex Soojung-Kim Pang argues that, amongst other drawbacks, 'overworking' negatively affects company performance because we're more likely to cut corners and to overlook small but crucial details. Putting in more hours doesn't necessarily help us get more done, or impress the bosses. In a study by Boston University's Questrom School of Business, managers could not tell the difference between employees who actually worked eighty hours a week and those who just pretended to.[49] Sometimes, working too hard even makes us sick. A study by the National Bureau of Economic Research (NBER)[50] showed working long hours actively caused health problems, increasing employees' odds of depression and heart attacks. Meanwhile, multiple studies by the Finnish Institute of Occupational Health have found that overwork (and the resulting stress) can lead to a range of illnesses and disabilities, including depression, diabetes, impaired memory and heart disease.[51] Britain is far from immune. In fact, British workers put in two and a half weeks more work per year than the average European, and half of our workplace absences are caused by stress, anxiety or depression.[52] A survey by Future Forum Pulse in 2023 reported that 42 per cent of workers admit to burnout[53] – an all-time high – with women under thirty most affected. It's no wonder that there's been a pushback by young women against ambition culture in recent years, from the trend of 'quiet quitting' to TikTok's #lazygirljobs.[54]

If healthy people are becoming ill because of the daily grind, it is not hard to imagine that people who are already living with chronic conditions could be hurt by the pressure to keep up at work.

Natasha Lipman, who has Ehlers–Danlos syndrome, worked a staff job as a journalist for the BBC until it took too much toll on her health. 'I'd been having a flare-up for about five or six months and I was really struggling to write and do my actual job. My pain and fatigue levels were extremely high. I found myself just staring at the screen trying to will words to come out and they just didn't. I ended up taking sick leave for seven months, and during that time I thought a lot about what I wanted to do in my life and how I was living. Nearly all of my energy went on work (and my side projects which are also, technically, work) and I didn't have any kind of balance. It wasn't sustainable and something had to give. At the same time, they shut my team down at work and I wasn't offered a role that was accessible.

'All I ever wanted to do was work. I spent most of my formative years as a young adult with my health getting worse and worse and leaving every job and opportunity that I had. It really hit my identity hard. I didn't know what it meant to just "exist", especially as I was seeing all my friends start to build lives and careers while I was stuck in bed. But now I'm older, I've learned I don't have to push my body to try to keep up with the healthy people around me. Because I can't.

'Leaving my job and then my freelance career has allowed me to not just think about work but to be able to help around the house and to think about hobbies and reading and resting. It was emotionally extremely difficult at first, but now I feel like I have a life outside of work. I'm now slowly getting back into "work" through volunteering in my local community. I've noticed benefits to my mental health, stress levels and overall ability to function physically throughout the day. I know I'm in an extremely fortunate position in that my partner earns enough for us to live on, so we could afford for me to take this step. That's not the case for everyone.'

As Lipman found, there are benefits to re-evaluating your workload but there are often hoops to jump through to get there. Society isn't set up for people who can't work or who work less – not just in the cultural messaging we receive but in the practicalities too. If you need a long break from your job, you'd better have a boss willing to let you take it. If we can't do regular or paid work, we have to find another way to pay the bills – whether that's a spouse, wading through the benefits system, or selling a kidney (unless you're taking time off because of your kidneys – pick an organ to flog that would get a good price is my only advice).

Navigating this maze is only made more complicated by the fact we often don't get a choice in entering it. For many disabled or chronically ill people, leaving or staying out of work isn't so much a decision we make than a situation that was forced upon us, either by our bodies or a system that too often doesn't support workers with health conditions. It's natural to be deeply affected by this. The loss of a career – be it one you had or one imagined – can feel achingly significant, not least in a world that puts such value on a person's profession. There is a grief to it, really, a mourning not only of the experiences we miss out on, or the balance in our bank accounts, but part of our identity with it. In some ways, falling ill or disabled is a (quite mean) lesson in just how much self-worth we place on what we can do, and just how insecure a ground that is to bet ourselves on. Or to put it another way: when the people at the party ask what I do for a living, what if I have no answer? Who am I then?

Not being able to do paid work means Evie Torrance, who has ME, chronic Lyme disease and migraines, has often felt judgement – both from herself and other people. 'If I tell people I'm a twenty-something disabled adult living at home with my parents, I'm immediately placed as "low" on the social ladder. However, if I then tell someone that I'm an author and have written two books, I immediately get placed back on the "worthy" list. But I am just as worthy today if all I had done up to this point was survive. I am just as worthy if all I had done was get through, day by day. Our worth is innate; it's not tied to anybody or any job or anything else. Every day, I have to learn this. Or, to be precise, I have to unlearn this. Every day, I have to redefine my idea of success. All the while constantly being told that my definition of success is not the "right" one.

'When people ask me what I do for a living now, I tell them I'm a part-time writer and full-time healer from chronic illness. I'm content with this answer, and it's taken me years – four, to be precise – to work out how to phrase it. But I would be lying to say I still don't find it hard.'

Josie George, who has ME, PoTS and chronic pain, is able to work reduced hours as a writer and artist but still wrestles with comparing herself to others. 'I've often really struggled with this idea that I must "keep up" with my non-disabled peers. I end up feeling inferior that I can't do as much as them and frustrated that my achievements always take *much* longer. It's easy to feel like I'm always behind and that everyone else is always better than me in some way. But I've learned to counter this by realizing that my differences are actually my strength. By being different and having to work in a different or slower way, I automatically create work that is unique and really special. My body and the way I have to live means that I see things differently. I have different thoughts. I produce different writing and art and say things that other people aren't saying. That gives me an edge! In a weird way, it makes you stand out from the crowd. All those people going faster are all conforming and competing over the same things in the same way, but you get to carve your own path. If you lean in to that and do what only *you* can do, that can be really powerful.'

When I fell ill, I found solace in work. It was like I was retaining a small piece of me, even as my body and life changed. I feel lucky it has remained one of the few things I can still do, at least in some form, but it is not easy. I sometimes wonder what more I could be achieving if I didn't have to deal with the bullshit my body (and an ableist world's reaction to it) throws at me on a daily basis. Could I in fact have cured cancer by now if I didn't have to spend sixteen hours a day in bed? (No.) In writing this book, my biggest concern was not my ability to think of the words to write but that I was in too much pain to sit at a desk to type them. That is objectively massively annoying. But I know the frustration also came from the (internal?) pressure to keep up with colleagues in similar fields, as well as – perhaps most painfully – the potential that I knew sat in me, if only my body would set it free. It is draining to have to dedicate 20–90 per cent of your

attention (varying percentages available) to simply functioning, not least when you are trying to reach the same
goals as everyone else: a fabulous career, big-money promotion, basic hygiene. I'm not going to pretend there is
a magic solution to any of this. I'm not going to suggest
that positive thinking can untangle the entire capitalist
system. Your to-do list is already long enough. But I will
say that we can question some of the ideas around work
we have been told are gospel, and reconfigure a version
of 'working hard' or 'doing enough' that is not only more
accurate – but better for us. Learning to dismantle some
of that expectation – to question where it comes from
and whether it is actually serving us – is perhaps the most
useful work we can ever do.

Part of this, I think, is redefining how we are told to
perceive 'work'. Talk about work and we still get the image
of an office and a pay cheque at the end of the month.
But this doesn't describe a lot of women's lives, or credit
all the contributions we make. As the old feminist adage
goes: there is no such thing as a woman who doesn't work,
just a woman who isn't paid for her work. Women are still
predominantly the ones doing the majority of childcare,
housework, and looking after elderly relatives. For disabled
women, there's often more work on top, from volunteering
in our community, advocating online for other people with
our health conditions, or just going to medical appointments and remembering whether we've taken our pills (or
just think we've taken our pills). That's work.

Besides, the idea that a disabled person has to complete some form of employment as a precursor for being seen as worthwhile is pretty troublesome. There's a popular saying that minorities have to work twice as hard to get half as far in their careers and there's certainly truth in that. The structural inequality we've seen in the last three chapters – from inaccessible education to lack of adjustments in the office – means disabled women often have to put in more hours, more tears, more ingenuity and still struggle to keep up with our non-disabled peers. That's not fair and it needs to change. But I can't help but think the feeling we have to 'keep up' is part of the problem. Maybe victory doesn't always come from forcing our bodies to do twice as much as other women who are dealing with half as much. Maybe sometimes it's about recognizing that getting half as far is enough. That we can stop entirely. It is a hard-earned realization that we have inherent worth as human beings, but it is one to repeat over and over – whether we are disabled or not. Our value is not defined by our output, just as there is no to-do list that we must tick before we can be granted approval. Feel frustrated at the impact disability and ableism is having on your career if you need. Let all the emotions out – anger, jealousy, sadness – and write it all down if that helps. But if other feelings – feelings of shame or guilt or embarrassment – rear their head, I hope you'll pause. I hope you'll remind yourself that there are count-less ways of contributing in this life and 'success' and 'prod-uctivity' take many more shapes than the non-disabled box we are forced to fit in. I'll start. It is OK if you haven't got your dream job. It is OK if your health means you can't work right now. If you've never had paid work. If you never will. It is all right if you're wearing yesterday's pants and you're considering sniffing them and giving them a whirl for tomorrow too. Rest is not failure. Sometimes, health is a full-time job.

As this chapter has shown, climbing the career ladder can come with particular challenges for disabled women – whether that's discrimination in getting hired, unequal pay, gaining modifications in the workplace, or stepping off the ladder entirely and leaving work. At the same time, we have seen the talent that disabled women are already bringing to swathes of industries and that – with support and our rights in place – we can often enjoy the same career highs as anyone else. It would be natural to look at our non-disabled colleagues and compare ourselves, or to hear our friends talk about their new promotion and feel a tug of sadness amongst the pride. A lack of ambition is not a symptom of any known disability, just like even the wobbliest of bodies holds on to its dreams. But keep on. Others aren't having to cope with the present you are, so don't pressure yourself to create the same future either. Do what you can with what you've got. I'd take a bet you've got so much more inside of you than you think.

Body Image

'I see [my body] as a glorious and intricate machine that I don't understand but praise daily for what it does do for me, rather than resent what it doesn't do.'

— Jameela Jamil

I'd been in bed a year when I thought it might be time to put a bra on again. From my teens onwards, I had loved fashion, and I think in some ways my disability encouraged that. If I felt self-conscious about my body, a blow-dry was an easy boost. If I felt judged by those who only saw the wheelchair, styling an outfit was freeing self-expression. Also, I have incredible taste. When I fell ill, that outlet vanished. Suddenly, I barely had the energy to clean my teeth, let alone put on a face of make-up. What had long been a key part of my life had overnight floated into the past. Dresses hung unworn in my wardrobe, foundation gathered dust in its box. The loss felt heavy, as if a ten-pound weight was physically tugging at my waist. I thought about it constantly and at the same time hardly at all. I suppose I had new priorities. When you're struggling to breathe, how you look doesn't tend to register above how you feel.

And yet I would be lying if I said that I hadn't been affected by the way my health has altered my appearance over the years. If it feels confidence-lifting to get a haircut and put on your best-fitting dress, it naturally feels confidence-zapping to be sat in jogging bottoms with your unwashed hair in a bun. This isn't just about how I look but I suppose a sense of who I am. In the ups and downs of chronic illness, few milestones have felt more moving than the days I have been well enough to get dressed up again. There is a magic to it: wriggling into an uncomfortable pair of jeans and the way mascara smells when it sets. In those moments, I have felt closer to my old self again than any other, as if I had rented myself out from a fancy-dress shop. Maybe that's patriarchal pressure that sends the message that a woman's worth is defined by her looks. Maybe it just feels nice to be washed and dressed. Even a chimpanzee likes to lick herself clean.

We don't really hear about this. Look at the solely non-disabled models featured in fashion mags or brand campaigns and it seems society believes disabled women have little interest in their appearance, as if disability precludes the butterflies of choosing a jumpsuit for a first date or buying a skirt for that new job. But the – entirely obvious – truth is, having a disability or health condition does not stop us from caring about how we look (or, like any other non-homogeneous group of women, not caring in the slightest). In fact, I'd say we have *more* to think about than most. If you're dealing with illness or disability, you're likely having to watch your body change in front of you: some added flesh, a bumpy scar. If you need to start using a disability aid, it can mean getting to grips with another way of looking different – and everyone else's opinions about it. Even getting clothes to fit can be a challenge if you're disabled, whether that's the lack of adaptive fashion or the fact inaccessible shops mean we can't always get in the building to buy them. At the same time, mainstream body-image movements based on 'what your body can do' can feel alien to disabled women whose bodies may be struggling to do the basics. It turns out that having a positive body image might take more than putting a bra on.

'What you lookin' at?'

Here are the rules of being a woman, as I understand them. Be confident but not *too* confident. Sexy but never slutty. Be slim but not thin. (Unless thin is 'in' again so do check your calendar.) Have a healthy glow. Smooth skin. Light is preferable, of course. Red lips. Big eyes. No wrinkles. But don't be vain. Every woman since the beginning of time has been handed the rule book of how to look – and promptly been told they are doing it wrong. For disabled women, that's especially true. By nature of being disabled, our bodies typically don't conform to society's patriarchal beauty standards. Whether because of genetics, illness symptoms or medical treatment, disabled bodies are often not the same as other women's. It is not just that our bodies don't always *do* what other women's do, it is that they don't necessarily look like them either. We have scars, curved spines, or shorter legs. We have missing limbs, patchy hair, or smaller muscles. We have extra flesh, medical tags, or burns. By merely existing, disabled women challenge the norms of what a woman 'should' be like. It is not so much that we throw out the rule book of womanhood, but smash it, pulp it and use it as kitty litter.

Historically, societies have long recoiled at the sight of disability. From the 1860s onwards, a number of cities in the US made it illegal for persons with 'unsightly or disfiguring disabilities' to appear in public. The last piece of legislation – known informally as 'the Ugly Laws' – was repealed as recently as 1974.[1] In our own country, 'freak shows' saw people with visible disabilities siphoned off from mainstream society and used as entertainment.[2] Famed throughout the nineteenth century but still touring as late as the 1960s, fairs featured 'midgets' or individuals with 'deformed bodies' as a means to exploit the public's fear and mockery of disability. Over sixty years later, disabled people in Britain may no longer be put in the circus but our appearance is still othered. Flick through fashion magazines and it's unlikely you'll see women who are visibly disabled. Scroll Instagram and the biggest accounts are typically white, slim, and non-disabled. In the few times that popular culture does permit disabled women to be open about our bodies, it is often labelled as 'confessional' or 'brave'. The implication is that freely speaking about or showing our bodies is, at best, unusual and, at worst, worthy of pity. The message is always the same: that it is the norm for disabled bodies to be hidden away from view.

In contrast, non-disabled bodies are held up as the ideal form. We have seen this particularly in recent years with the advent of online wellness culture, in which celebrities and influencers sell elite bodies as the optimum goal, and with it, the belief that with the right choices (and purchases) – a juicing diet, hot yoga, the odd vagina crystal – you too can glow with health. In our culture, health is not viewed as just a physical benefit but an aesthetic to be coveted, a kind of lifestyle brand exclusively for women with the right genetics. Here, being healthy is not a bit of good luck but a moral virtue – a physical sign of purity, discipline and glamour. It is not caused by structural inequality, like housing, healthcare or wages, but praised (or blamed) squarely on the individual. Of course, elevating the appearance of 'healthy bodies' only serves to further marginalize disabled ones. If good health is aspirational, bad health is repulsive.

This doesn't just mean that disabled women are excluded from society's conception of what is beautiful, but that we are held up as a symbol of what is ugly. To be a disabled woman is to routinely be told by the world that we are made wrong – that we are unattractive, unfuckable, or simply invisible. While all women can suffer from the pressure of the 'ideal body', disabled women are uniquely stigmatized for 'failing' to meet these standards. If a woman being fat or unshaven is a challenge to patriarchal rules, a woman who dares to show off her scars or stoma is an abomination. In a society in which a woman's purpose is still to be conventionally attractive and fertile, women who are sick or disabled are seen as an offensive subversion. This revulsion at female disability manifests in multiple ways – even attempts to exclude disabled women from public spaces. In 2019, the BBC reported on the online harassment of disabled journalist Melissa Blake[3] who posted an article on the US election only to receive thousands of comments about her accompanying photo. Blake, who has a genetic bone and muscle condition that affects the mouth, face, hands and feet, was told she was 'too ugly for selfies'. In response, Blake shared three photos of herself on X.

The internet may have opened up new ways to judge women but it has long happened in the offline world too. Few of us with a visible disability have managed to walk down a street without at some point being stared at. As a wheelchair user, it's always been part of life for strangers to stare at me, mouths slightly ajar like carp. Without saying a word, staring at a disabled woman sends a clear message: how our bodies look is weird or repulsive and we don't really belong out of the house with the rest of you. In a culture that says disability and chronic illness prevent a woman from living a full life, it is almost confusing to see someone who 'looks disabled' taking part in 'normal' activities that are thought to be the preserve of non-disabled people. For some, seeing a disabled woman laughing at a festival or browsing in a department store is like spotting a fish on land. They just aren't meant to be there. If I think about it, I have always found myself stared at more in places associated with fun or sexuality, such as a nightclub or beauty salon. It feels as if people are shocked by someone like me even being in those spaces, their gaze seemingly physically unable to ignore the oddity of a woman with a broken body paying for a drink at the bar.

At the more extreme end of the spectrum, being visibly disabled in public can lead to abuse. Disability hate crime in England and Wales is alarmingly prevalent, with more than eleven thousand incidents of verbal or physical abuse reported to police between April 2021 and March 2022[4] by disabled people (though this is thought to be an underestimate due to barriers to accessing justice). The charity Changing Faces says reports on hostile behaviour towards those with a visible difference, such as a scar, mark or other condition, have been on the rise in recent years. Reports of hostile treatment by the public increased from a third of people with a visible difference in 2019 to more than two in five in 2021.[5] While there is no specific data on the experiences of disabled women, campaigners such as Dr Amy Kavanagh report[6] women with disabilities often face a toxic blend of sexist and ableist treatment, from being touched by a member of the public without consent to having their mobility aids pulled away. Simply 'looking disabled' in public can be enough to get you harassed.*

After suffering a life-changing acid assault, broadcaster Katie Piper was left blind in one eye and with extensive burns, including throughout her face. It led her to suffer deeply difficult changes to her body image as well as verbal abuse from the public. 'Before I was burned, I was really into make-up and fashion. In my late teens, I went to beauty college. Then I lost my hair. The front of my head was shaved for the surgeries, and the back fell out while I was in a coma. When my hair was growing back, I grew a fringe and styled it a lot while it was short. It's not vain to say that my hair changing and growing over the years really shaped how I felt about myself. Initially, I wore a plastic face mask for two years to help my scarring heal. I had very purple skin. Strangers reacted by shouting at me in the street, asking me to leave shops. Men would wolf-whistle from behind when they could just see my long hair or shouted, "Oi, blondie!" and then when they saw my face, they'd say "monster" or "freak". I refused to hide away. I educated people about why I looked this way.'

---

* Being visibly disabled can be all the harder if you're marginalized in another way. If you're trans, you might have to worry about looking 'feminine enough' to go in women's toilets without trouble, just as you're emptying your catheter. If you're black, your boss could be criticizing your natural hair as 'unprofessional' when seeing clients, as well as asking you to cover up your scars.

Against this backdrop, it's unsurprising that disability can have a significant impact on how women feel about our bodies. A groundbreaking survey by the House of Commons Women and Equalities Committee in 2020[7] into body image found disabled people are at higher risk of experiencing negative emotions around their appearance. Some 71 per cent of people with a disability reported feeling negative or very negative about their body image compared with 60 per cent of people without a disability. This resulted in people with disabilities experiencing a range of emotions about their appearance, from feeling ignored, judged, to isolated. Smaller-scale studies consistently show disabled women in particular struggle with confidence around our bodies. One study published in *Sociological Focus* asked twenty-one physically disabled female students about how they saw themselves and what they thought the ideal woman looked like. Researchers found that many of the women interviewed believed the ideal woman to be incompatible with having a visible disability. For example, some reported that they imagined the ideal woman as 'not misshapen'.[8]

Model Jillian Mercado can nowadays be found on the runway, but for years she struggled to feel confident about her thin muscles caused by muscular dystrophy. When Mercado was young, she heard negative comments about her disability, including being told that her condition was 'some sort of curse'. It had a significant impact on her emotional wellbeing to the extent that she struggled to leave the house in the summer unless she was covered up. 'I was extremely scared of going outside in a short dress or short shorts. In the days of New York where it would get up to ninety-five degrees in a super-hot day, I was wearing a long dress or long jeans, refusing to show my legs. I still have very skinny legs but back when I was younger I thought they were the most ugliest thing you can think of. [I didn't know] that this was not something that I came up with, this was a thought that society gave me. I thought that if I did wear those shorts people were going to point and laugh, that I was going to get called names. [I didn't understand] that those negative thoughts were preventing me from actually enjoying a simple pair of shorts.

'I remember that one day I was tired of disliking a part of myself that I had no control over. One extremely hot summer I told my younger sister that I was ready to try to wear shorts outside. She told me that there was no rush, and that if I was scared, to just walk around the block and see how it feels. So I did. One block became two, two blocks became three hours, and after a whole day of being outside in the park enjoying the beautiful weather, I remembered that I had this fear of these exact [shorts] and nothing happened. My fear prevented me from loving my body. Since then I wear my short dresses and short pants even knowing that I still have my skinny legs. It's a slow progress and there are times where I am hesitant but it has definitely helped my confidence. It's so much easier now to wear exactly what I want without having any fear of what others might think of me.'

For Piper, it was a combination of friends, specialist make-up, and therapy that enabled her to slowly rebuild her faith in her body image. 'Discovering beauty and medical products for my scars really helped with my confidence. When I was first scarred, I tried loads of different products that didn't actually work. That felt really hard psychologically. Nowadays, I feel able to leave the house without make-up most days. I post on social media no make-up photos. That didn't come overnight. There were many bad days, many good days. I spoke to a psychologist, people I loved, and people who had facial differences like me. Some people think that confidence can come from appearance – looking good, being thin, being pretty – but it doesn't. I've learned that confidence is a lot about self-acceptance. Accepting ourselves as we are, rather than aspiring to be like somebody else. If we have life-changing events happen to us, especially something like disability, we can learn to love ourselves a little bit more. There is so much beauty in trauma, the imperfect, the unfiltered. I can say I now love the skin I'm in.'

When photos of pop star Selena Gomez in a bikini emerged in 2023,[9] the images quickly went viral. Gomez, who has lupus and has previously undergone an emergency kidney transplant, was seen grinning as she swam in the sea off a luxury boat – but to many onlookers, there was a reason to be miserable: she had put on weight. What wasn't obvious from first glance was that Gomez's size had fluctuated due to the heavy medication she regularly takes to help her lupus. No one could technically 'see' her disability but it had nonetheless altered her body and other people's attitudes to it.

Many of us will know how this feels. 'Invisible disability' is an odd – and telling – term, really: it describes how non-disabled people see our disabilities, not our own experience of them. Invisible (sometimes known as hidden) disabilities are very much visible to those of us who have them. It's hard not to notice you have Crohn's disease when you're hugging a toilet bowl. That's the same with our body image, I think. Disabilities that are technically 'hidden' can still alter our appearance, from putting on weight from medication like Gomez, pulling out patches of hair due to anxiety, to using a cane on a high-pain day. These changes don't even need to be physical. If you have to give up or cut back on work due to health problems, you lose the disposable income to treat yourself to that new dress. When you're regularly poked and prodded at medical appointments, it can feel as if your body isn't yours any more. Being affected by all this isn't superficial – it can go straight to our sense of identity. Watching our bodies change can feel like watching ourselves change, and in a way we have little or no control over. Add to that other people's opinions and the toll can feel achingly heavy. Evidence backs this up. Research shows health conditions that are 'hidden' have an impact on how we feel about ourselves just like visible conditions do – and interestingly, some suggest they can even have a greater impact. A 2019 study into the impact of disability on body image[10] found that those who had a disability that was not observable by others – for example, a mental health condition – actually felt more negative about themselves and their body than those who had a disability that was easily observable by others.

This is familiar to author Luce Brett. When Brett developed incontinence after childbirth in her early thirties, she became acutely self-conscious. 'I suddenly had to be so prepared, either wearing pads or protection or carrying spare clothes with me, and tailoring outfits so they were less likely to make a noise or bulge too much. Black leggings became my standard uniform. I was nervous of smelling or leaking so badly that other people would notice. Of making a mess on a chair or public transport. The stuff of nightmares. Incontinence requires a brutal devil-may-care pragmatism when it comes to styling, but also, you know, your sex life, how you have fun, your day-to-day life, and the resilience to accept you're having to spend so much time, energy and vigilance thinking about knickers and pads. I'd have to be talking about urine burn and prolapses and pad-use and pessaries and then pulling on my damp black leggings and marching back out into the world as a mum of tiny kids, a partner, a working professional, and just act like I was *absolutely fine* and no I didn't have wee on my coatigan.

'I think I'd absorbed a million deeply harmful messages both about women's bodies and illness being shameful but also birth injuries and incontinence being something trivial that just happened to older ladies. It was a hell of a thing, being so young and feeling like everything – the leaflets, the information, the products – was designed for someone else. I couldn't believe it was happening to me. I had to take a deep breath and realize that this was my life, this was my body, and without sounding twee I had to find a way to make the best of it. And sometimes that feels mindful and intentional and wise, and other days it involves too much smoky eyeliner and a hefty heap of my best bullshitting to get me through.'

As someone who gradually lost her vision throughout her childhood, musician Andrea Begley can only remember what she looked like until her early teens. It's given Begley a unique relationship with her body image: while her disability doesn't alter her appearance, it does mean she can't check in on it. 'Most people stereotypically expect visually impaired people to not really care much about how they look. After all, we can't see it, so why make the effort. In one sense, I'm immune from the picture-perfect world of social media that many others find so challenging. This does not mean I don't suffer from my own form of comparison issues, though. I think I'm so used to not seeing myself now that I rarely think about it, but it does become difficult to totally remove that innate desire to look in a mirror and see what is looking back at you. Ninety-nine per cent of the time I think little of it and life just runs on, but sometimes I do let the thought in. Like most people, I can have good body days and bad ones. I can't see the wrinkles or the greys, so sometimes that's a blessing and sometimes it's so frustrating, when you can't tell if your top is the correct shade of blue or if your hair is sitting the way you like it.'

For writer and small-business owner Rosie Fletcher, it was medication that quietly altered how she felt about her body. When Fletcher fell ill with ME and several autoimmune disorders, she went on a diet 'presumably for want of a proper hobby'. But when her steroid medication led her to gain weight, Fletcher began to confront the pressure she felt to be thin. 'Three years after I got ill, I logged everything I ate in an app and restricted my calories. In any circumstance, only eating two-thirds of the calories you need is a bad idea but I had chronic fatigue. My life was entirely dictated by a lack of energy and I was purposefully not putting enough fuel in the tank. If I couldn't be useful then I might as well be beautiful, no matter how useless I became to achieve it.

'As time went on, I began to eat more. Around the time I gained weight, I started on steroids. Side effects of all stripes can be really distressing because, even though you know you're taking the medication for good reason, changes in how you feel in yourself can be so jarring. It feels like pure vanity to complain about it. I think we brush off "weight gain" as a small-fry side effect but "no longer adhering to socially imposed beauty standards" is not the easiest pill to swallow. Pun intended. Now, I'm the biggest I've ever been and I'm the most comfortable I have ever been in my body. I take my body on long walks and don't show it the calorie counts on packets any more. I spotted my little back rolls in a changing-room mirror for the first time and just giggled at the *Drag Race* reference instead. I only feel bad about myself when I try on clothes that don't fit. So I bought cute new clothes that do.'

'Aren't you young to be using that thing?'

'You're too pretty to be in that chair, love.' I imagine most of us who use a disability aid have received this sort of comment at some point in our lives, typically from a sweaty man at 1 a.m. outside a Walkabout. Whether it's a hearing aid, a white cane, or a wheelchair, there is something about using a disability aid in public that often triggers such a reaction. 'You're too pretty to . . .' is said as if it is a compliment but, of course, it is code for something altogether more insulting. They are saying that being disabled and attractive are two mutually exclusive things. They are implying that a visible sign of disability would 'ruin' an otherwise good body (which is the only thing a woman is for, naturally). They are saying that disabled women should hide our health needs in order to look 'normal'. Being a woman with a disability aid is much like being in one of those 1990s high-school movies where the nerdy girl takes off her glasses and is suddenly deemed beautiful enough for the jock.

We know all too well that women, disabled or not, are routinely told to adapt our appearance and behaviour to fit sexist standards. That we should be as small as possible. That we are not meant to take up space. But this takes on an added level for disabled women, few more so than those who use disability aids. In a culture in which women are raised to 'not make a fuss', and illness is still regularly seen as shameful and ugly, women with disabilities are routinely told to conceal any signs of it. This attitude is not just consigned to drunk men in pubs. Think of the viral wedding clips where the bride is lifted out of her wheelchair to walk down the aisle to a row of celebratory comments. Or the family member who crops your cane out of the group photo 'because it ruins it'. If you're disabled, you must give non-disabled people the courtesy of pretending you are not.

I don't necessarily think of this as a sign of meanness or deliberate bigotry but a reflection of how the wider public is told to see disability. We might call it the non-disabled gaze – that is, that non-disabled people often perceive disability as a tragedy or weakness and therefore associate being visibly disabled as a negative that's best erased. One result of this is society's skewed attitude towards disability aids. While, by definition, an aid actually makes a person's life easier, many non-disabled people nonetheless still see using one as something worthy of pity. This manifests in expressions of sympathy – 'it's such a shame you're in that chair!' – but also apparent praise too. How many of us with a visible disability have been doing an errand only to be told by a stranger we are 'so brave', as if a wheelchair user deserves the Victoria Cross for queuing for a sausage roll at Greggs. Such sentiments can often be well-meaning, but dig a little deeper and they are not actually about the disabled person – they are about deferring to the feelings of the non-disabled bystander who feels awkward or sad to see signs of disability on an otherwise 'normal body'. In the viral video clips in which a bride gets out of her wheelchair, for example, the moment is framed as more about the delight of her loved ones (and strangers on the internet) at her 'overcoming the shackles of disability' than her own feelings. To the non-disabled gaze, the ultimate moment of a woman's femininity – her wedding day – cannot possibly co-exist with her using a mobility aid. The celebration obviously has good intentions but the question becomes: what are we actually applauding? A body that doesn't look disabled? And if that, then why?

It's not only that we're often told we shouldn't use a disability aid – sometimes, we're accused of not even needing one. Anecdotally, it's common for disabled people who use a disability aid to be doubted by strangers, as well as loved ones or even medical professionals. Over the years, I've heard of countless ambulant wheelchair users yelled at in the supermarket 'for faking' when they stand up from their chair to reach a shelf. Or stoma users – whose health condition isn't visible – chastised when they come out of an accessible toilet, because 'that's for real disabled people!' Such stigma can be especially prevalent for those of us with a fluctuating disability, where being seen using a cane one day and walking unaided the next is judged as 'proof' we don't really need one at all. This of course happens to men too but often takes on a sexist edge when it means policing women's bodies, where disability aids are simultaneously cast as 'too ugly' for a pretty girl to use and a precious object only *other* women deserve. Such prejudice is particularly levelled at young disabled women, who are frequently judged for not fitting the stereotype of being 'old enough' to need assistance. This is only exacerbated by the fact disability accessories are still primarily sold by companies aimed solely at elderly people, simultaneously robbing young customers of stylish aids that suit their age and perpetuating the myth to the wider public that young disabled women don't use them. In this context, it becomes quite normal for a complete stranger to declare, 'You're too young to use that cane.' (Babe, tell my joints that.)

It's no wonder that in this culture many women admit to being reluctant to use their disability aids in public, even if it means suffering through worse symptoms or not leaving the house. In some ways, it is the ultimate act of controlling a woman's appearance: shaming her to give up a disability aid that makes her feel better. The viral collaboration between Lady Gaga and Hollywood legend Liza Minnelli at the 2022 Oscars was a case in point. Minnelli, who was reportedly experiencing back pain at the time, sat in a wheelchair throughout[11] the presentation. Media coverage later said the actor had been 'sabotaged' and 'forced' into using the wheelchair by organizers and had wanted to sit in a director's chair instead. 'You know, I want to look good,' Minnelli reportedly said backstage when offered the wheelchair. 'I don't want people to worry about me.' Her fears weren't exactly irrational. Headlines about her appearance characterized the actor as 'frail', while social media users debated whether her shaky conversation with Lady Gaga meant 'she wasn't all there'.

The incident shows clearly how the messages society sends about disability aids don't just impact non-disabled people's views. Rather, toxic ideas about disability unknowingly filter through disabled people's heads, like a carbon monoxide leak. Terms like 'internalized sexism' and 'internalized homophobia' – to describe how minorities can subconsciously accept or project the stigma they face – are common nowadays but 'internalized ableism', though less mainstream, is just as powerful. Think of it as an inner voice that sends self-defeating, generally shitty messages about having a disability. This can produce a range of harmful results – even women struggling to refer to themselves as 'disabled', despite experiencing debilitating symptoms for years. Some might be encouraged to believe they don't 'deserve' to call themselves disabled because others have it worse, as if disability were graded on a curve. Others may feel shamed by society's prejudices about disability. These messages often crop up when we start to need a disability aid too. That using an aid is 'giving up'. That we don't really need or deserve one. That it desexualizes or makes us 'infirm'. In many ways, this inner conflict is not just about how we look with a disability aid but what it means to use one.

As a BBC broadcaster, Nikki Fox proudly sits in her scooter on national television each week. But she wasn't always so confident. When Fox first began to struggle to walk in her early twenties due to her progressing muscular dystrophy, she felt uneasy about starting to use a mobility aid. 'I guess it's like a different way of viewing yourself. That you're suddenly really disabled because you're using a mobility aid. Which is ridiculous. If anything, I looked "more disabled" bobbing around walking. My head and neck jerk back, you don't want to see that! Comparatively, I look practically elegant sitting in my scooter. But did I feel "more disabled"? Did that make me a failure? If someone else asked me that today, I'd say, "Of course not!" but honestly, that's how I felt at the time. Plus, I never really knew how my disability was meant to develop. They told my dad that me and my sister [who also has a muscle weakness] would use a wheelchair when we were ten and we walked until we were twenty-five. But is that right? Should I have kept pushing on? You think: did I cave in?'

It's normal to have these sorts of reservations. It's OK to have mixed feelings too. I remember when I got my first electric wheelchair when I was eighteen. After a decade of using a manual chair, I couldn't propel myself any more and had to rely on adults pushing me around school. I was excited for the independence and the simple but remarkable ability to move from one place to the next myself. But I was self-conscious too. The new wheelchair took up more space, and as a teenager who wanted to blend in, moving around with battery power felt the equivalent of holding a sign up that said, 'LOOK AT ME.' I didn't want to be noticed. I didn't want to need to be. In time, though, I adjusted. I realized I could be grateful that the technology existed and wish sometimes that I didn't have to use it. I could feel frustrated with the chair and feel liberated by what it enabled me to do. Maybe you're having similar thoughts right now. It's possible to miss going for a run while being happy your cane lets you walk. It's OK to be confident that a hearing aid helps you talk to strangers and feel self-conscious they may stare at it. Equally, acceptance isn't linear. You can have cracked Zen-like peace one day and then be pissed off all over again the next. Feelings are complicated things, not least when you're trying to deal with yours but everyone else's too.

Like most things in life, the hardest part is often the start. The first time your new boyfriend sees your catheter as you undress. The pep talk you give yourself one Tuesday in front of the mirror before trying out your crutch in

Sainsbury's. This is something medal-winning Para-lympian Stefanie Reid MBE, who started to use a pros-thesis after becoming an amputee at fifteen, knows very well. 'For the first few years, you would never catch me in shorts or skirts. I ordered a cosmetic leg painted skin colour because I was uncomfortable "looking disabled". I thought the way to be successful was to learn to walk so well that I fooled people into thinking that I wasn't an amputee. I made friends in university that two years in still didn't know I was an amputee. Part of me didn't want people to feel sorry for me. I just wanted to get on with my life. But part of me also felt like it was something I needed to hide. It was like I was trying to fool people into thinking that I belong. That I wasn't something "other". But the problem wasn't them. It was me and how I felt about myself and about disability.

'Getting back into sport sparked a change in me. People didn't feel sorry for me when they saw me run. They thought it was cool. And I didn't mind them staring. In fact, I ordered my running leg in hot pink – there was definitely no missing it! My carbon-fibre leg is awesome. People should stare at it. I would stare too! That was when I stopped ordering my everyday prosthesis in painted skin colour. I decided to stop trying to turn the leg into some-thing it was not. It wasn't a real leg and it never was going to be. I decided to go with a carbon-fibre cyborg look. It became an exclusive fashion accessory that no one else could have. I stopped worrying about how I compared to other people. The best thing I can be is me and be me to the extreme.'

For actor and screenwriter Genevieve Barr, who is deaf, it was turning her hearing aids into a brightly coloured accessory that helped her embrace them as a teenager. 'When I was thirteen, I had ear moulds in rainbow colours and I would paint the plastic backs with nail varnish. I was not a fashion person but I did not like beige, and as they were beige, they needed sorting out. I grew up in the Spice Girls mania of the 90s – every teenage girl wanted to be loud and kickass so my hearing aids were too. When I was sixteen, hearing aids changed from analogue to digital. Suddenly the battery power went from incredibly loud and crackly to quiet and robotic. That had a really profound impact on me. I think I stayed quiet for two weeks. The bubble popped – growing up, I'd casually assumed my hearing aids were a replica of everybody else's hearing. It really upset me. Then I adjusted, as we always are expected to do. I couldn't live without my hearing aids. They're my armour and I rarely take them off. It's always been that way. But taking them off at the end of the day – the silence before going to bed – it's an oasis.'

The idea that someone like Barr would see her hearing aids as precious armour runs counter to how we're encouraged to think. When someone says they're getting their first disability aid, it's often viewed as a sad moment. This person could have been wincing in pain to walk round the office or been shut away at home because they were too weak from lack of nutrients. But still, starting to use a cane or a feeding tube would likely be greeted with pity. This attitude isn't extended to any other solution or tool in life. No one pulls a sad face when someone uses a washing machine instead of struggling to rinse their jeans by hand. Using an aid to help our bodies is no different. A feeding tube makes you strong enough to start going out to see your friends again. Having a cane means you can get to that meeting without being exhausted from unnecessary pain. It says a lot about how warped our view of disability is as a society that such events could be seen as anything other than a positive. Culturally, we have already normalized people wearing glasses to help their eyesight; there is no rational reason this attitude can't be extended to other pieces of health equipment. For all the doubts and insecurity, to many disabled people, disability aids are not suffocating – they are freedom. Starting to use one is not a tragic thing to pity. It is liberation to celebrate.

For Fox, years on from worrying about starting to use a scooter, she's thankful for all it's given her. 'Before I had my scooter, I was so restricted that I had to plan everything down to the letter. If I couldn't find a parking space less than a few feet from the pub entrance, I wouldn't be able to go at all because I couldn't walk that far. I remember when I first sat in the scooter. I went to work [as a TV runner] and the producer asked me to go and get him a sandwich and I thought, Wow, I can actually do that. I'm in a scooter. I can go wherever I want. That freedom outweighed any negative thoughts I may have had. I no longer live a restricted life. My scooter gave me independence. For that, I love it.'

Even dogs have more clothing options

The first sign is the flash of panic across their eyes. Over the years, I've come to understand there is no worse question to ask a shop assistant than 'Do you have an accessible changing room?' It is up there with 'How would you like to be murdered?' and 'Could you check out the back?' It is not their fault, I know. It is not their fault that a grey-haired man in head office decided a multi-million-pound company didn't need to spend a few hundred quid on a wider cubicle that would fit a wheelchair. It is not their fault that the world, in its creaking curtain rails and low benches, is built for non-disabled bodies. But then, it isn't mine either.

'Special-occasion shopping' is always the worst; the weight of expectation dragging like a plastic security tag. Over fifteen years later, I still remember the futility of looking for a graduation dress. A friend and I headed to a high-street shop, unreasonably priced formalwear draped over two floors. Womenswear was downstairs – 'Men are too lazy to use stairs,' the shop assistant explained – but there was no lift. 'Don't worry,' she reassured me, wheelchair users could use an alternative changing room: the stock cupboard. I'd like to say this was the first time I'd been asked to strip off in a cupboard, but as a disabled woman who likes fashion, it's been a semi-regular occurrence through-out my life. I still think of the shop assistant in the depart-ment store who breezily walked in on me half-naked as she searched for stock. I couldn't blame her. It was, after all, a stock cupboard. Still, with no other option available yet again, I bit my lip and agreed to the latest offer: I took off the rails a short gold dress that smelled like sequins and acceptance. And I shut myself in the closet.

Changing rooms aside, clothes shopping has never been the easiest task for me. When you spend the day sitting down, standard designs too often bunch, dig in, or ride up. Buying a dress as a wheelchair user is much like being Kim Kardashian at the Met Ball: you may feel like Marilyn Monroe standing up but you can barely breathe sitting down. Back in the closet, it took two minutes for me to realize that the dress in question was getting stuck as I yanked it on. It turns out stock cupboards are not designed for stretch-ing and I flailed aimlessly for what felt like eternity. There I was. Squatted next to a mop and bucket, sequins pulled halfway down my arse. I had never felt more glamorous.

This sort of experience is depressingly common. Despite anti-discrimination laws in the UK giving some rights to disability access, many shops on the high street are still inaccessible for disabled consumers. The UK Disability Survey in 2021 found shopping to be the most inaccess-ible type of business on the high street, with 78 per cent of disabled respondents saying they had frequently been unable to access or had extreme difficulty accessing shops and shopping centres.[12] The growth of online retail over the last decade has opened up access for some disabled people, but for others, it means more frustration. Some 98 per cent of the million most-visited web pages did not meet accessibility standards, according to the same survey.[13] The result is missing out entirely; 69 per cent of disabled internet users click away from sites with barriers, such as low-contrast fonts and images without alt-text for visually impaired customers.

The scale of this exclusion is vast. A government audit of more than thirty thousand shops and restaurants in 2014 – still the biggest ever of its kind in the UK – found there to be 'shocking' access on the high street for disabled people.[14] They reported a fifth of shops had no wheelchair access and only 15 per cent had hearing loops for shoppers with hearing loss. Two-thirds of retail staff had no training in how to help disabled customers, while less than a third of department stores had accessible changing rooms. Shopping while disabled is essentially fantastic if you enjoy being very uncomfortable, paying over the odds, or flashing.

As a scooter user, broadcaster Nikki Fox has struggled for years to access shops as well as suitable clothes. 'In or out the scooter, I've never found clothes shops very accessible. The changing rooms are so small and I take ages to get changed. The mirrors are shite. I've always ended up having to buy the clothes, try them on at home and then take anything back. Nowadays, I just do it online. It takes out the faff.

'When I started using a scooter, I had to kind of learn how to choose clothes again. Clothes sit differently when you're sitting down. Your posture changes. I felt like I essentially lost my shoulders. And I loved my shoulders. At the same time, my body was changing. When I was walking, it took so much effort to get around that I could eat anything. Turn up to a McDonald's drive-thru and order nine hash browns. Once I was using the scooter, I put on two stone in practically two weeks. I'm not hung up on weight, and I hate that we are as a society, but it does get to you. In the end, I decided, y'know, I'm going to have to work out how to style this disabled tush in a scooter. I've still got great tits! They're bigger, actually.'

Fox's experience highlights a key point: if you're a disabled woman, it isn't just a matter of struggling to get in the shops – if you do get inside, there may be few clothes that you can buy. If you have a sensory-processing disability, you might find traditional waistbands uncomfortable. If you struggle with dexterity, buttons and zips can be impossible. This is not a niche issue. A study by Primark and the Research Institute for Disabled Consumers (RIDC) in 2024 revealed a massive 62 per cent of disabled shoppers said it was difficult to find clothes they feel happy and comfortable in.[15] And yet adaptive fashion – that is, clothes that are designed specifically to adapt to various disabilities – is still rarely sold by mainstream brands. Walk into any high-street store and there will be clothing for specific consumers, be it maternity, plus size or petite. But there will be no similar range for disabled customers. As Stephanie Thomas, a congenital amputee, put it in her TEDx talk on the issue: 'We have more clothing in stores for dogs than we do for people with disabilities.'[16]

After becoming a wheelchair user in her late teens, broadcaster Sophie Morgan found herself faced with the challenge of styling clothes that were designed solely for women standing up. 'When it comes to my body, I struggle with self-acceptance as much as most women. Using a wheelchair permanently means that clothes often don't fit me very well, so I've had to undergo a lot of trial and error to find what works. It's a constant work in progress! I've learned to style and dress myself so that I feel more confident when I'm at work presenting on TV. I use control underwear or corsets to help me sit straighter and hold in my paralysed tummy and I have lots of tattoos all over my body to cover my scars or make my body more colourful and beautiful.'

For social entrepreneur and broadcaster Shani Dhanda, being much shorter than the average woman because of brittle bone disease means she has to buy clothes that are too large for her stature. On top of the underrepresentation of Asian women in the fashion industry, this deficit in clothing options made for her disability has 'massively' affected Dhanda's body image over the years. 'When I was younger, I found being both disabled and Asian combined to affect how I felt about my body. I was never told I was beautiful, I never felt desired, and I never saw anyone like me – or South Asian women generally – in the beauty pages.

'I'm the height of a three- to four-year-old. I live in a world that isn't designed for me and struggle to find clothes. And when I do find something, I have to pay to cut half of it off! It even overshadows certain situations where I should be excited to do something but I'm more worried about what I'm going to wear. Last year, I attended the BAFTA awards ceremony as I judged one of the categories. I was really excited to go, but that feeling of dread washed over me as it came to thinking about "what am I going to wear?" It was short notice so I [didn't have] enough time to get anything custom-made. [In the end], I [took] a heavily sequined jacket I'd previously bought from ASOS [and] sewed it together to make it look like a dress. It was really heavy, and I was really hot in it . . . I constantly have to settle with what works over what I actually want to wear.'

Recent years has seen progress in adaptive fashion as a way to solve these dilemmas, helped in part by the extra options that have been born from the growth in online retailers. In 2016, Tommy Hilfiger launched one of the world's first mainstream collections of adaptive clothing – from adjustable hems, easy-open necklines, to one-handed zips, each alongside the brand's signature red, white and blue palette. Two years later, IZ Adaptive, stocked by Zapped, the Amazon-owned global retailer, launched their own range, including trousers with horizontal pull-tabs at the side (enabling wearers with dexterity conditions to pull them up without having to grip), as well as coats with magnetic fastenings. By 2025, high-street jugger-naut Primark was launching a 49-piece adaptive product range – thought to be the biggest ever collection by a mainstream retailer[17] – with Marks & Spencer announc-ing knickers designed for stoma users just a few months earlier.[18] At the same time, the UK has several emerging options: from Unhidden,[19] which includes clothing for people who have ports and monitors on their body, to Adaptive Fashion UK, an online space dedicated to disa-bility-friendly clothes.

And yet even with these strides, fashion designed specific-ally for disabled people is still almost exclusively confined to online, small (often disabled-led) boutiques, and prohib-itively high-priced. The 2024 study by RIDC found that although 77 per cent of disabled shoppers said adaptive clothing was essential to, or significantly improved their quality of life, only 25 per cent said they currently wore it due to barriers including affordability and accessibil-ity.[20] As Dhanda – who acted as a consultant on the Primark clothing range – puts it: 'I've not yet shopped [adaptive fashion]. There's only one [range] I can think of that offers anything for me, and that's so expensive even for basic items.'

I can't pretend that this surprises me. The cultural prejudices around disabled women and fashion I spoke of at the start of the chapter don't exist in a vacuum – they directly impact how companies treat us. If designers believe disabled women don't enjoy fashion like other 'normal' women, then there's no point in making us clothes. If clothing brands don't think disabled women have careers and a disposable income, then it doesn't matter to them if their shops aren't accessible to us. There's a reason you rarely see a fashion ad campaign with a model sitting in a wheelchair. In fact, disabled customers are ready and willing to be prime consumers: one estimate puts the spending power of disabled people and their families at £274 billion per year,[21] with high-street shops thought to be losing £267 million a month due to lack of disability access.[22] It wouldn't be an act of charity for clothes shops to become accessible – it's good business.

For all the scale and complexity of it, it would be remarkably easy to make the fashion industry more accessible for disabled women. To provide one changing room that is slightly bigger to accommodate a wheelchair. To put some adapted clothing next to the 'petite' and 'plus size' rails. To avoid strobe lighting to help people with seizures stay safe or install a hearing loop to enable Deaf customers to hear. To do . . . something. Anything. There is a wearying normality to inequality after a while, where you convince yourself that wading through boxes of cabbage to enter through the goods entrance or trying on a top in the middle of the store protected only by display rails* are perfectly standard ways to be treated. I won't pretend that making fashion more accessible would single-handedly improve disabled women's body image but I can't help but think it would be a start. Imagine going into your favourite store and feeling like you belong there – seeing an accessible entrance that welcomes you, clothes on the rails designed for you, and changing rooms built for you. Imagine what it would feel like to go into a shop to buy a graduation dress and not be asked to change in the stock cupboard, but be treated just like everyone else. I don't think that's actually too much to ask.

Just think positive

There's a scene in *Sex and the City* in which the four friends sit naming the things they hate about their bodies. Charlotte detests her thighs, Miranda her chin, while Carrie gestures knowingly to her nose. Samantha, meanwhile, remains silent. Waiting for their friend to do her feminine duty and join in with the self-flagellation, the three women stare at Samantha. She shrugs. 'I happen to love the way I look.'

* Both actual things I've done.

I suppose I'm a Samantha. I can't say that I 'love' the way I look but I don't have any desire to insult it. I've never spent more than a minute thinking about the parts of my body I don't like. I've never been on a diet. I recoil whenever I hear the phrase 'guilty pleasure'. This is partly because I really like bread. But I think it is also a product of having a disability. Growing up, I would often notice the shame that non-disabled women carried with them about how they looked. Classmates would point to their boobs and bemoan how 'flat-chested' they were. Older colleagues would go to lunch and wince at the offer of dessert. Their bodies, their perfect bodies, always had 'something wrong', even as they ran and danced and sang. As a physically disabled woman, it felt like watching the owner of a Porsche worry about a tiny scratch on the boot.

I decided a long time ago to be kind to my body. I would come back from every chest infection at school grateful for each breath of air. Yet another fortnight of uni spent stuck in bed with a minor cold only reinforced how carefree I was once I could finally leave the house. While my non-disabled female friends paused over a third piece of pizza, I'd willingly gorge. I was not immune to the hang-ups that come from living in a sexist society – and I more than understood why they felt that worry – but I suppose I was gifted with what you might call a different perspective. I knew what it was to have a body with problems, and a bit of extra fat around my tummy did not make the list.

Research suggests I'm not alone in this. While – as this chapter has shown – disability can negatively affect our body image, it can also have the reverse effect. One study[23] into the body-related attitudes of disabled women actually found having a disability lessened their hang-ups. The disabled women interviewed seemed to worry less about small changes in weight and shape than their non-disabled peers, and to have what the researchers called 'an enhanced sense of their own robustness'. Another study found that disabled women who are new mothers may have greater acceptance of their changing body image than new mums without disabilities. Researchers found that while non-disabled mums were likely to take non-aesthetic qualities like bodily function and independence for granted when their bodies stopped conforming to strict appearance standards, disabled women were able to appreciate these aspects of body image as important.[24]

Actor Jameela Jamil, who has Ehlers–Danlos syndrome, can identify with this. 'It's [my health that] actually made me look at my body in an abstract and surprisingly appreciative way. I see it as a glorious and intricate machine that I don't understand but praise daily for what it does do for me, rather than resent what it doesn't do. Of course there are frustrating days, but generally I maintain a sense of immense gratitude. I feel genuinely quite grateful for it. I think I would have died of anorexia had I not grown such immense respect for what a survivor this body is. I've decided it is an absolute legend and ultimately my very best friend who is doing what it can, however swollen and complex and painful it is, to help me achieve my dreams.'

For comedian Rosie Jones, having cerebral palsy has in many ways increased her sense of confidence over her body. 'I think my disability had a positive effect in terms of my own body image. Naturally, like most people, I could pick faults with my body. I'm too short, my tummy is too big and I have a mole on my forehead that I *really* dislike. But I've never felt the need to change my body to "fit in". This is because even if I were five inches taller, with a flat tummy and a moleless forehead, I'd still stick out like a sore thumb because I'd still be "the wobbly one". Having a disability gives you a bit of perspective when it comes to body image because, at the end of the day, I don't care what my body looks like; I'm just glad it works!'

Like Jones, I used to have a similar stance. As long as my body got me to work and the pub, I couldn't have cared less that my stomach wasn't flat. If I think about it, I didn't just give myself an extra slice of pizza because I had perspective on what really mattered – I did it as a 'thank you'. My body was doing so much for me, despite all its disadvantages. The least it deserved was some more cheese. But I know that when I fell ill, that mindset became less and less clear. When I was disabled but still able to do most things I wanted, I found it easy to be 'positive' about my tired muscles. By the time I fell chronically ill and was too fatigued to see friends, it was hard to imagine what function

I should be 'grateful' for. That becomes all the harder when we consider how an inaccessible society further disables us. Being grateful your body gets you to the office becomes more complicated when your bigoted boss passes you over for that promotion. Whether it is our disability itself or how society relates to it, there will always be times – many of them, probably – when, for all the positivity and pep talks, we feel weighed down by the restriction we face, like a shipwreck in the sea. Or to put it another way: it's one thing to like our bodies when they're working but what if they're not?

Mainstream body-image movements struggle to give answers to such dilemmas. 'Body positivity' – which advocates having a positive view of your body, no matter what shape or size – has gained a lot of traction in recent years. Originally created by black and fat women in the 1970s, it is in many ways a welcome riposte to a culture that teaches us from puberty onwards to pick ourselves apart with the language of cottage-cheese thighs, muffin tops, or Hula Hoop toes (fine, I made that last one up). And yet as a disabled woman, the narrative has always seemed a little alien to me. When your body is causing you so much pain, it is a tough ask to feel positive about it. Besides, the focus on appearance feels almost naive; a bit of extra fat or a few wrinkles barely register as concerns when you're struggling to get dressed. The way in which the body-positivity movement has been co-opted by thin white women online over the last decade has only felt more exclusionary. Conventionally attractive women declaring that they 'love their tummy rolls' is little help to those of us whose bodies genuinely challenge the status quo.

Meanwhile, 'body neutrality' – a concept based on acceptance rather than overtly positive feelings, often pegged on the body's abilities – has emerged as an alternative, but in some ways, such an outlook still feels intrinsically ableist. It is easy to be accepting of your body when you've just run a half-marathon; much harder when you're struggling to make it out of bed to the toilet. As writer Rosie Fletcher, who has ME, puts it: 'Body-positive [and body-neutral] mantras told me to focus not on what I looked like but what I could do; think how far those fat thighs take you, what your wobbly arms carry. My thighs took me to the kitchen for breakfast and then back to bed for the day.' It is not as if the outside world helps by sending warm fuzzy messages to counter any of this. When anything, from the workplace, education, basic infrastructure, healthcare, to popular culture routinely shuts disabled bodies out, society provides neither a positive nor even neutral view of the way ours work. It is openly hostile to it.

I can't help but think, as I poke my tired skin, that disabled women need alternative ways to relate to our bodies. If traditional movements like body positivity and neutrality can feel excluding to many disabled women, what strategies can we look to? If hyper-positivity feels oppressive, is there still a way to feel confident? If we can't rely on function to feel good about our bodies, what can we focus on?

For broadcaster Sophie Morgan, who was paralysed as a teenager, her strategy is to practise gratitude for when her body works and acceptance when it doesn't. 'I've needed several horrid, invasive reconstructive facial surgeries over the years to help me breathe but I've not had any cosmetic surgery. I can't justify the suffering I experience in a surgery solely in order to make me feel better about my appearance. It has taken me a while to realize that I have the power to choose how I feel about my face, and that it's best to choose to accept it than try and change it. As I've got older, my face is ageing now but I'm thankful I've made it this far. All my wrinkles and frown lines are signs I've lived a full life. I've chosen to accept the body I have and try to love it for what it can do, not hate it for what it can't. I might not be able to move two-thirds of it, nor can I feel anything below my chest, I've no ability to tone or shape my stomach or legs, and I've got incontinence due to being paralysed, but my body is all I have and it has enabled me to do so much. My body might not "work" like other people's but it functions well enough for me to be able to live my life to the best of my ability, and for that I am so grateful.'

After years of resenting her body's painful endometriosis, journalist Lara Parker began to practise radically loving it when it suffers. 'For a long, long time I hated my body. And I think so much of this stemmed from my pain and my illnesses. I hated my body for letting me down. I hated myself for allowing it to fail me. I hated what I saw in the mirror because what I saw was a sick fucking body that didn't work. But I started going to therapy, and in therapy I learned all about reframing things. I reframed the idea that my body was fighting *against me* and finally realized that my body is fighting alongside me. My body is doing the best it can to fight against my illnesses *just like I am.* After that, I began to try and celebrate my body more. I started being nicer to myself. And now? I love myself . . . I throw love at myself so aggressively until I have no choice but to give in and remember that my body is the vessel that carries my soul and it deserves my love and appreciation, even on the hard days. Especially on the hard days.'

Achieving this sort of self-acceptance is not an easy task, but I reckon it is one worth trying – and then trying again and again. My own relationship with my body may have changed with chronic illness but I think I've managed to find peace with it. Most days. I can be frustrated at what it can't do or upset at what that means I've lost while being immensely proud of everything it does do. It feels A Great Injustice that the people who are getting on day-to-day with (let's call them) difficult bodies, all while living in an ableist society, are shamed rather than celebrated for it. An Olympian privileged with optimum genetics may get the gold medal but have they ever managed to put deodorant on in a pain spike? Show me the way to the podium.

If you are struggling with how you feel about your body right now, I hope you're kind to yourself. None of this is easy and I'm not going to fill these pages with trite words that pretend otherwise. But next time you find yourself staring in a mirror and thinking a thought that is mean and niggling, I hope you'll pause for a moment. Because I can tell you without a doubt that you are fucking glorious exactly as you are, and that the best favour you will ever do yourself is helping your brain believe that. There are many ways that we can reclaim our bodies from illness or disability (and society's perception of it), each unique to the person: from finding community with other women who look like us, listing what we value about our body, to – my personal preference – hoarding so many pots of skincare that they have to be stored in a wardrobe. And yet at the same time, we should never lose sight of the bigger picture. It would be convenient to put the responsibility for disabled women's body image on to the individual, to suggest that if only we tried harder or bought the right products, we would be happier. But the onus should always be on challenging the ableism, sexism, racism, transphobia and fatphobia that runs through society. We tell women to 'love their curves' while algorithms sell them diet pills and shame. We call disabled women 'inspirational' for existing while endorsing a system that routinely questions their existence. Rather than blindly demanding disabled women love ourselves, perhaps it is time to ask why it is exactly we might loathe ourselves. Disabled bodies are not the problem, the way that the world relates to disabled bodies is.

As this chapter has shown, our body image can be significantly affected by disabilities and health conditions, and society's reaction to them. While anything from physical symptoms to the use of disability aids can alter our appearance – and how we feel about it – mainstream feminist body movements can feel excluding if you have a disability. Thankfully, we have also seen how disabled women are challenging these prejudices, and with it reclaiming our bodies and our confidence. I smile whenever I see women making these strides. The gastric patient on Instagram creating art out of her facial feeding tube. The paraplegic on TikTok healing from tattoo ink laced across her skin. And yet I can't help but think this is more than a matter of disabled women reclaiming ourselves – it's a matter of reclaiming space. Because none of this has ever really just been about how we look. It is about the ability to live freely. To walk through the world unencumbered by other people's narrow-mindedness and to trust we deserve to be there. To sit on a park bench in the summer heat in your favourite dress and feel the sunlight on your scars. No one has the right to take that away from you: no magazine, social media algorithm, or ex. In a world that too often teaches disabled women to hate our bodies, it is a radical act to love it. Or to simply quite like it sometimes.

Healthcare

'He turned to the other doctors and said,
"She just wants to be handicapped, doesn't she?
There's actually nothing wrong with her."'
— **Cherylee Houston MBE**

When I got sick, my bedroom curtains caught on fire. Except they didn't. It turns out the mind can play tricks when the body is going through trauma, and for me, that meant conjuring up imaginary flames. Like a particularly advanced pyromaniac. Two weeks after developing flu complications, I was in bed struggling to breathe or move. I had no idea if I would ever get out, or even what had put me there. In the early hours of the morning, my fear saw smoke billow up the windowpane. I can still remember the terror of becoming that sick, though it is muted and grey. It is a bit like they say about childbirth. Your brain provides a protective response that never lets you fully remember the pain, or you'd never choose to do it again. Except with illness, you don't get a choice. Or the compensation of an orgasm.

Looking back, I know now that the trauma I felt wasn't simply from being ill – but that I had no clear path to get well. When we are healthy, we tend to believe doctors fix you. We are told this from an early age. 'Tell the nice man where it hurts and he'll make it better,' your mummy says. Dress in the white coat with a stethoscope round your neck and you can cure every teddy of any disease. Within a few months of getting sick, I knew this was a lie. It wasn't simply that medics didn't know how to treat me, it was how they *treated* me. As both a woman and a disabled person, I have long come to know that accessing healthcare means facing a set of assumptions: that disability means having a lower quality of life; that I am incapable of making decisions myself; and 'difficult' if I politely push back. This has significantly increased since I became chronically ill. Over the last seven years, there has rarely been an encounter with a healthcare professional that at some point has not left me feeling small. Where I have not had to lobby to be listened to or to be seen as capable or fully developed. I have perfected a 'bit' where if a medic is particularly patronizing, I tell them I need to check my work calendar before making a new appointment. We both know that I am not actually just checking my availability, I am performing a role. The role is 'adult who has a life that matters'. I play with my iPhone for forty-five seconds and they wait, wondering if this is what a disabled woman should be like.

No one should need a 'bit' to receive healthcare. No one should be made to feel like they are less than a person when they just want to feel better. And yet patients with long-term health conditions consistently report receiving poorer healthcare than our non-disabled peers. Treatment for many chronic conditions can be elusive. Just getting a diagnosis is often an uphill battle. These barriers don't stop with our own health conditions. Disabled women and non-binary people even miss out on healthcare unrelated to our disabilities, from mammograms, smear tests, to dentistry. At the same time, there can be a dearth of support and advice available to help women with long-term health conditions learn to live with our symptoms. When the teddy and the plastic stethoscope are long gone, what is left is the uncomfortable truth: too often, those of us who are the very patients who need the best healthcare can end up with the worst.

It's all in your head

On the first night I couldn't breathe, I called an ambulance. The paramedic arrived an hour later, his Australian accent calmly puncturing the panic in the air. He placed a heart monitor on my chest and watched it bleep and crunk. 'It always does this,' he muttered apologetically, hitting the machine with his fist. The lines on the screen reassured us both I was probably not having a heart attack and I curled up in bed, hoping I'd wake up from the bad dream.

On the second night I couldn't breathe, I went to A&E. I was more tired than I had ever been and I wondered aloud if the two new events were linked. 'Exhaustion shouldn't affect breathing,' a consultant told me, as I gasped for air. My respiratory muscles, chastised for their wilfulness, went home. I didn't know it at the time but this mix of dismissal and ignorance would characterize my healthcare from then on.

Over the months that followed, I became my own detective. I knew I had recently been sick with the flu, that I hadn't felt right since, and that, logically, that must have been the trigger that led to a severe post-viral reaction from my already weak muscles. And yet to many medics I saw, it was assumed that any symptoms I was experiencing were purely down to my existing disability. Others spent their time disputing my symptoms, confused that my disabled body was behaving differently than other, 'normal' patients. There was no search for a diagnosis or investigation of my sudden fatigue and pain – just an assumption this was inevitable. As one GP put it to me as I sat on a ventilator, 'It might just be a decline in your disability.' I was given a prescription for painkillers and wished well, as I sat there wondering how exactly genetics change overnight.

I've received much excellent healthcare over the years. Smart, kind support from wonderful people dedicated to their jobs that I'll always be grateful for. It is very easy to talk about that, particularly in a country with a universal healthcare system that consistently needs defending from those who would dismantle it. What feels harder to talk about is the poor care. The long waits and botched diagnoses. The cruel words and dismissive tones. It feels almost sacrilegious, as if acknowledging the NHS's short-comings somehow means we don't support it or that minor-ities should just be grateful for any care at all. It doesn't help that disabled patients receiving unequal healthcare – whether that's in the NHS or private clinics, in the UK or elsewhere – goes against the essence of how society perceives medics. We would expect few people to under-stand and care about disability more than medical pro-fessionals. After all, they see it every day, don't they? But doctors and nurses are not immune from the social biases that affect how those of us with disabilities are seen, even if we wish they were. The prejudices and stereotypes that plague disabled women in education and the workplace exist everywhere, even in the place that is meant to help us: healthcare.

Research consistently shows that disabled people are viewed – and treated – more negatively by medical staff compared to non-disabled patients. A 2022 US study[1] saw doctors admit under anonymity that they treat patients with disabilities differently, including limiting their care or getting rid of them entirely. Doctors reported telling wheel-chair users they should go to a cattle processing plant or a zoo to be weighed, because their clinic would not accom-modate them, and lying to a new patient that the practice was closed. Many of the medics interviewed showed dehu-manizing and devaluing attitudes towards disabled people.

A specialist in one focus group said disabled patients took too much time, adding that they were 'a disruption to clinic flow', while another believed people with disabilities – who may require adjustments to help them access healthcare – are 'an entitled population'. This bias against disabled patients even extends to how valuable our lives are. As one academic paper in 2015 put it, healthcare workers often perceive individuals with disabilities as 'vulnerable', of low competence, or less value.[2] Staggeringly, another study in the US found more than 82 per cent of physicians believe people with significant disabilities 'have worse quality of life than non-disabled people'.[3] These attitudes have real-life consequences. A study by the Urban Institute in 2023[4] found disabled adults in the US were three times more likely than adults without disabilities to report unfair treatment in healthcare settings (32 per cent versus 10 per cent). About 71 per cent of those who experienced unfair treatment reported a subsequent disruption to their care, including delays (54 per cent) or not getting the care they needed (50 per cent).

At its worst, discrimination can even impact how long disabled people live. On average in the UK, the life expectancy of women with a learning disability is a shocking eighteen years shorter than for women in the general population.[5] It would be easy to assume this was largely down to lifestyle factors (such as the fact disabled people are more likely to live in poverty or have multiple health problems) but the data shows that many lives could be saved with equally good healthcare. The confidential inquiry into pre-mature deaths of people with a learning disability found that 38 per cent died from an avoidable cause, compared to 9 per cent in a comparison population of people without a learning disability.[6]

The coronavirus pandemic starkly unmasked this bias against disabled patients. As hospitals became inundated with Covid in the spring of 2020, the BMA set out guidance to ration treatment if the NHS became overwhelmed with cases.[7] The plan was matter-of-fact: in the event that ventilators were scarce, people who had an underlying health condition could have the life-saving equipment taken away from them – even if their condition was improving – with younger and healthier patients given priority instead. Meanwhile, the National Institute for Health and Care Excellence (NICE)[8] advised doctors to withhold treatment from patients scoring high on 'frailty scores' – including people with learning disabilities and autism – on the basis they needed support with personal care in their day-to-day life. The guidance was only pulled when disability groups threatened legal action. By 2021, rationing of healthcare was no longer hypothetical: England's care watchdog found disabled people – particularly those with learning disabilities – were given Do Not Resuscitate orders (DNRs)[9] when they contracted Covid, often without being agreed in discussion with the person or their family.[10]

As anyone who has ever developed worrying health symptoms knows, it is often an uphill battle to find out the cause. A survey by Global Genes found it takes an average of five years in the UK, and over seven years in the US, to accurately diagnose a rare disease.[11] The study found that, along the way, a patient typically has to visit up to eight medical professionals (four primary-care and four specialists) and receives two to three misdiagnoses. Even common conditions can go undiagnosed for years. Research shows symptoms of multiple sclerosis (MS) may commonly be missed for up to five years before the right diagnosis is made.[12] Meanwhile, people with bipolar wait for an average of 13.2 years before they are diagnosed, and often spend years receiving treatment for the wrong condition.[13]

Some delay in diagnosing an illness or disability is of course understandable, particularly for conditions that are still medically misunderstood. But one group are notably managing to get diagnosed quicker: men. Women are more likely to have chronic health conditions[14] across the board[15] but at the same time are less likely to receive a timely diagnosis. A large Danish study found, on average, women were diagnosed four years later than men across seven hundred illnesses, including cancer, diabetes and ADHD.[16] Research backs this up across multiple different conditions. It takes an average of twelve months for men to get diagnosed with Crohn's, an inflammatory gut condition, compared to twenty months for women.[17] When it comes to autism, women typically receive a diagnosis several years later than men[18] and have their symptoms wrongly attributed to other conditions. Men are diagnosed with the connective tissue disorder Ehlers–Danlos syndrome on average in four years. For women, it's sixteen.[19, 20]

Let's call this Medical Groundhog Day – where women experiencing debilitating long-term health problems must go back and forth to the doctors on repeat to try and get answers and help. A major survey by the Department for Health and Social Care in 2021[21] of over 100,000 respondents in England sums this up starkly: more than four in five (84 per cent) women have experienced times when they were not listened to by healthcare professionals. This manifested in their symptoms not being taken seriously when they first made contact with GPs or other health professionals, and in them having to persistently advocate for themselves to secure a diagnosis, often throughout multiple visits over the course of months and years. If they did manage to get a diagnosis, the study found women's preferences for treatment are often ignored.

It all adds up to mean disabled women are in many ways up against double institutional bias in the healthcare system, simultaneously facing ableism and sexism from doctors that too often sees their symptoms and concerns dismissed.

Professor Bethan Evans, a senior lecturer in Human Geography at the University of Liverpool, who has ME, anxiety and depression, explains these attitudes go back centuries:

'There's a long history of women being disbelieved or disregarded in medical practice in Western medicine. Women's bodies are traditionally viewed as unruly and emotional – think of histories of diagnoses of women's health problems as "hysteria" or "malingering", for example, or the stereotype that women have weaker wills. Frustratingly, that's still often the case today. Women's accounts of their experiences of pain, illness and other symptoms are often considered untrustworthy and are more likely to be seen as psychosomatic or "all in their head". This is even more so for women of colour, and trans and non-binary people. Conditions that are more common in women are less likely to be seen as serious.[22] At the same time, some chronic conditions, such as ME, fibromyalgia, autoimmune disorders, and more recently long Covid, are particularly dismissed or disbelieved and even classified incorrectly by medics as mental health conditions.'

The stats back this up. Research by Chronic Illness Inclusion in 2021 showed that a third of women surveyed in the UK had waited more than ten years for a diagnosis – and that before receiving their current diagnosis, four in five respondents had their physical symptoms attributed to various psychosocial causes by healthcare professionals, such as anxiety or stress. About a half had been given psychological therapy – not for a diagnosed mental health condition, but to treat their undiagnosed physical symptoms.[23]

It is hard enough to feel unwell but even harder to feel unwell and not know why. Without a diagnosis, it can be more difficult for us to access treatment options or help to manage – often worsening – symptoms. This can in turn take a heavy toll on our lives: from having to stop work to withdrawing from friendships and relationships. Dr Katharine Cheston, formerly a researcher at the Institute for Medical Humanities, Durham University, who previously had ME herself, says the hunt for a diagnosis can have a vast impact on women. 'Many women have told me in interviews that they'd consulted multiple different doctors – sometimes over a period of many years – in the hope of finding one medical professional who would listen to them and treat them with respect. This can be an exhausting and extortionate process, as those who can afford private healthcare are set back significant amounts of money in their search for better care, while those who can't afford this are left with even fewer options. As well as financially, being disbelieved can have a damaging impact psychologically. These women are often repeatedly made to feel their symptoms don't matter by the medical professionals they encounter – as if they're unimportant, as if they're nothing. In turn, many of these women express feeling as though they themselves don't matter: that they've been "written off". Women naturally internalize negative comments made by their medical professionals – or friends, family, colleagues – and in the absence of any other explanation for their symptoms, they blame themselves for it.'

A medical test coming back 'normal' is typically a moment to celebrate but anyone with undiagnosed long-term symptoms knows it can make things even harder. Cheston says that many women report this is the point when medical staff's attitudes to their treatment options noticeably change. 'At best, they describe healthcare professionals losing interest, or discharging them from their clinic. At worst, a number of women have told me that they feel as though medical professionals have judged them, disapproved of them; that their "unexplained" symptoms mark them out for, and perhaps even encourage or condone, mistreatment. They describe being made to feel unwelcome in healthcare spaces such as hospitals, and even being made to feel unworthy of the care that medical professionals provide them. I've spoken to a number of women who have expressed that they have not sought help from medical professionals – even, in one instance, where a woman developed new, worrying symptoms that she knew were suggestive of cancer. They have been let down so many times that they don't feel there's any point wasting their limited energy, or even that they have been made to feel so deeply ashamed that they don't feel they deserve help.'

Actor Cherylee Houston MBE first showed signs of EDS as a child but didn't receive a diagnosis until she was twenty-four. In the intervening decade, she was repeatedly shamed by doctors who didn't believe her. 'I started with symptoms at age eleven – pain and fatigue. I was diagnosed with growing pains, then arthritis. Then my parents started to be told that I was making it up. We went to many doctors. I spent most of my teens in different plaster casts or tuber grips. I was in a lot of pain all the time but by the time I'd hit sixteen I stopped telling anyone as no one believed me. My parents were told to ignore me if I was saying I was in pain as I was "looking for attention". When I moved to Manchester for uni, I was excited about new specialists. This doctor examined me and then got me to walk across the room; I limped and dragged myself across. He said, "Wait here," and came back with a couple more doctors and told me to do it again. He turned to the other doctors and said, "She just wants to be handicapped, doesn't she? There's actually nothing wrong with her." They thought I was making my walk up. Now I know my bones were dislocating.'

Looking back, Houston says not being believed made her 'much less vocal' about her disability in later life. 'I didn't really tell anybody about being in pain until I was in my mid-twenties and I never really spoke about it to people I didn't know until my mid-thirties. I used to take a leaflet about Ehlers–Danlos to hospital with me as evidence for doctors. I haven't had a specialist EDS doctor for twenty years so I often see medics who are unfamiliar with the condition. I think I still do have health PTSD from that time [when I was undiagnosed], I get trauma around certain health situations. But I know that my experiences have also taught me to be a great advocate for myself and to do my own research. I'm no longer quiet about my disability. I'm proud about what it has taught me and I'm vocal and honest about it.'

It took journalist Lara Parker five years of scouring message boards and medical websites to match her symptoms, as well as navigating several doctors and invasive procedures, to get a diagnosis of endometriosis. Like Houston, the experience has had a lasting impact on Parker's mental health and the way she navigates the healthcare system. 'The journey to receiving these diagnoses is something that I am still trying to work through these days. It was very traumatic for me, and something that has had a negative impact on my mental health in the years following. It's extremely difficult to live in one reality where you *know* something is going on with your body, and then to be told repeatedly that you aren't actually in reality but imagining this all as test after test comes back negative. It's been very hard to get to a place where I can advocate for myself and trust myself to know best. So much of Western medicine places doctors on pedestals that they simply do not deserve. It should always be that the patient is the expert of their own body and then go from there.'

Parker's experience shows clearly how there can be a power imbalance to medical appointments. As we saw in the chapter on careers, there are still few doctors who have a disability themselves. In almost four decades of healthcare, I have never seen a consultant who wasn't a man. Tackling this discrepancy is one of the long-term changes that could make a real difference to the healthcare that disabled women receive: from more women and disabled people being encouraged to go into medical research; practical adjustments to increase the number of disabled people in medicine; to compulsory disability and equality training for medics who aren't necessarily disabled themselves. In the meantime, though, there are strategies we can have in our armour for our next medical appointment.

Trishna Bharadia, health advocate and a visiting lecturer in patient engagement at King's College London, who herself has MS, says a good starting point to advocating for better care for yourself can be to find out what the standard of care *should* look like. 'So check out what the approved road to diagnosis is for a particular condition, according to your circumstances. For example, seeing which tests you should be getting and which type of healthcare professionals you should be seeing, within certain time periods. In the UK, this would involve looking at the NHS website and NICE guidelines, which you can also find online. Knowing your patient rights within the NHS is also key, and you can find this is set out in various documents on the gov.uk website. If you're not getting what you should be, then print it out and take a copy of the guidelines to your appointment – it shows you've done your research and know what you should be getting.

'If you're not happy with the response, remember that you're entitled to a second opinion. For primary care, that might mean requesting an appointment with a different GP in the practice – if this is being made difficult, then again, speak to the practice manager. For secondary care, this would involve going back to your GP and requesting a referral for a second opinion to a different hospital. If you don't know where to go for a second opinion, it can be worth talking to other patients. Join a Facebook group for your condition, speak to the national charities for your condition – many will have helplines – and ask if there's any local groups you can join. That way you'll be able to ask for recommendations from other patients. If all else fails, you have the right to make an official complaint. To voice any concerns or grievances through an official route, speak to the practice manager for primary care or Patient Liaison Service for hospitals.'

If you do decide to raise a formal complaint to the NHS, there's help out there. In every area in England, you can get support from what's called an Independent Health Complaints Advocate – someone who can help you understand the official complaints process, explore your options, write letters to the right people, and navigate meetings. While it's important to know our rights, and the support available to exercise them, the reality is that taking on a full-blown complaint can feel overwhelming, especially when you're unwell. It's easy to tell disabled women to 'complain' when they face discrimination, but it's us who have to find the energy to do it.

Sarah Deason, from The Advocacy People, a charity that helps advocate for disabled people, who herself has chronic migraine, says thankfully it's often possible to lobby for changes to our healthcare informally without going down the official route. 'Many issues are caused by misunderstandings or poor communication that can often be put right once the problem is explained. If you feel you are able to, you can speak to a member of staff who has been directly involved in your care and treatment or ask to speak to their manager. This is often the quickest way to put things right and prevent issues from getting worse. When discussing your concerns, be clear and straightforward. Don't be afraid to say what has upset you. Avoid aggressive or accusing language, put your concerns politely but firmly. And ask if you don't understand what's being said. Consider asking a friend or family member to help you prepare and perhaps go with you to appointments or be there when you speak to someone. They can prompt you, take notes or ask questions you haven't thought of. Make sure you share with them what you want to say so they can advocate for you. Think about how you'll react if you're not happy with the response from the healthcare professional. You might want to ask why and whether there are any alternative options. You might want to ask for a second opinion. It's OK to say you want to take time to think about what they have said and make a decision.'

Dr Deepti Gurdasani, a clinician and senior lecturer at Queen Mary University of London, who herself has the digestive condition ulcerative colitis and endometriosis, has experienced both sides of the doctor and patient line. 'In an ideal system, disabled women's suffering would be seen and acknowledged by healthcare workers. But in reality, this often doesn't happen, so we need to shift our goal to be about simply getting help. It is much easier for healthcare professionals to dismiss distress and emotion, especially coming from women and marginalized groups, so try adapting your phrasing. For example, "I'm in so much pain I can barely get dressed every day" is easier to dismiss than "I'm only able to get dressed on one out of seven days a week because of my pain. What can you do to make this better?" This is a way of presenting your problem list to the healthcare professional which then presents them with a set of issues they need to figure out solutions for.

'Be very specific about what you want – for example, a referral to a specialist, or a focus on how to combat a particular symptom. Prepare for the appointment and set out objectives of what you want to achieve, and work towards these goals very specifically rather than leaving them to the medic to raise. If you can, attend with a friend or partner who can witness what happens. If not, you also have the option of looking into recording your consultations so you have a record to refer to. Long term, though, there needs to be retraining of healthcare professionals. The onus for advocacy shouldn't be on the disabled community or on brown or black women. It should be on medics.'

The drugs don't work

It is August 2019 and I am wincing in my wheelchair. Pain has been a constant companion since the flu complications and I am meeting with a nurse to ask what I should do. 'Would seeing a physio help me learn to sit up comfortably again?' I ask. 'We haven't had one since the community funding was cut,' she says. 'Anyway, physios aren't for people like you.'

It is November 2019 and I am touring medical departments who have never met one another. A fatigue clinic. A pain clinic. Lung-function team. GP. Neuro team. Treatment for a long-term health condition feels like the equivalent of wanting to cook a Sunday roast – if you have to go to the beef shop, and also the carrot shop, the potato shop, the Yorkshire pudding shop, and then the gravy shop. It would be a lot easier if all this was in one place. After a year of chronic illness, I realize that – no matter how ill you feel – the healthcare system does not volunteer a treatment plan. Instead, I slowly become my own medical team. Asking for a consultant, googling symptoms, waiting a year for an appointment. I become on a first-name basis with the secretary of my GP surgery. I know hers and she dreads mine.

It is March 2022 and my breathing is getting worse. Unable to get sufficient support from the NHS, I speak to a kind private physiotherapist who is going through my treatment options for free. I discover there is such a thing as a respiratory physio and it is standard practice I should have one. Wondering whether the NHS can afford to fund them, I text my respiratory nurse asking if one is available. It turns out my team had one all along. I resist asking her: if that was the case, why wasn't I referred four years ago or when I called repeatedly to report worsening fatigue and pain? I resist going completely mad.

If you have a long-term health condition, it can sometimes feel like you're attending a different healthcare system than your friends and family – and not just because while your mates in their twenties and thirties will probably go years without ever seeing their GP, you see the inside of the local hospital more than the pub. To most patients with a short-term illness or injury, 'healthcare' means having your concerns believed and getting effective treatment;* to those of us with longer-term conditions, it too often means languishing on waiting lists and being left alone to cope with our symptoms. This is partly because chronic conditions are still often misunderstood or under-researched compared to common and short-term issues. Modern medicine is pretty remarkable at dealing with acute problems like a heart attack or stroke but much less advanced when it comes to treating chronic illnesses or disabilities. But we know the disparity in care is also due to a range of other complex factors, in which a cocktail of lack of joined-up services, overworked

---

* If you are a person of colour or from another minority background, though, this is not necessarily the case. More on this soon.

staff, ableism and ever-shrinking resources combine with underfunded research to leave disabled women too often in limbo without adequate treatment. Trying to get care for a broken leg is very different than trying to get help for unexplained pain.

The evidence backs this up. Research by academics at Cardiff University[24] found people with disabilities in the UK have significantly worse access to healthcare than patients without disabilities, with transportation, cost and long waiting lists being the main barriers. Tellingly, women reported worse access to healthcare than men, across all categories. A survey by the Chronic Illness Project in 2021 shows a similarly bleak picture for disabled women; only 17 per cent of women with long-term health conditions reported they felt supported by healthcare services meant for their disability.[25] Meanwhile, a survey by the disability charity Sense highlighted how poor access can block disabled patients from getting the treatment they need; over one in five people with complex disabilities said that healthcare staff 'rarely or never' meet their needs,[26] while the same proportion reported that their medical appointments 'rarely or never' happen in a way that is accessible to them.

Things get no better when you look at the treatment of specific health conditions. A survey of people with EDS about their healthcare experiences[27] found one in five (22 per cent) had a lack of trust in their healthcare provider, with over 40 per cent holding negative expectations for future healthcare. Elsewhere, a survey of people with neurological conditions highlighted the struggle in even getting regular appointments: over a quarter (26 per cent) said they last had a meeting with a consultant more than a year ago. Over one in twenty[28] said that they had never seen a neurological specialist.

This has only been exacerbated in recent years in the UK as the NHS has faced increasingly tough staffing shortages and a lack of resources. With funding squeezed[29] at the same time as need has grown, waiting times in England have hit a record high.[30] The knock-on effect for patients and staff alike has been as brutal as it was predictable. A YouGov poll in 2023[31] found 71 per cent of NHS staff who have direct contact with patients said they now have too little time to help those in their care. Nearly three-quarters – 74 per cent – of doctors, nurses and other staff who have worked in the NHS for at least five years said the quality of care they had been able to provide had got 'worse'. While many non-disabled people have struggled to access care in recent years, the impact of inadequate resources often hits harder for those of us with long-term health conditions. We are, after all, the people relying on the health service the most. Just look at mental health. Some 1.9 million people were on the waiting list for treatment from mental health services in England in 2023,[32] plus a further 8 million who couldn't get a referral because they weren't deemed unwell enough to qualify for support.[33]

This is all too familiar for journalist Hannah Jane Parkinson. Parkinson, who has bipolar and ADHD, has been receiving treatment for mental health conditions on the NHS for over a decade but has repeatedly struggled to get the care she needs. 'I used to think about moving to the US at some point and the two things that stopped me were the egregious healthcare system and the absurd obsession with guns. Now the situation in the UK with the NHS [feels little better]. I've been on many waiting lists for months, and in some cases two years, to see psychiatrists and psychotherapists. And I am someone who has a fifteen-year history of mental health difficulties, two diagnoses, has been sectioned before, and a history of suicide attempts. When I was under a section, the police took me to a hospital in central London, where I remained in a room, by myself, for twenty-four hours while the support workers and bed allocators tried to find a bed for me. There have been times when I couldn't even source my medication, because I couldn't get a GP appointment in time, and supply-chain problems sometimes mean pharmacies run out. I've recently started therapy again on the NHS after [being on] a two-year waiting list. In the meantime, I've spent thousands of pounds on private medical care, basically all of my savings. Because otherwise I'd probably be dead. It isn't something I can easily afford [but] I know I am very lucky indeed to be in a position to do so.'

You don't forget the morning your medical team refers you to social services. For two years, my fatigue had made it impossible to attend hospital appointments in-person – a particularly unhelpful development of acquiring low energy, next to choking on a chip at least once a week (and then proceeding to carry on eating the chips). The Girl Guide mentality that comes with a lifetime of disability means I'd worked out decent alternatives: regular lengthy remote appointments with doctors and other medics, and home visits for blood tests and breathing checks. Still, there had always been a sense of disbelief around it, a tense exchange and a tone from healthcare staff that said, 'I bet you could leave the house if you tried.' At one point, a respiratory nurse called my GP to explain they could send me hospital transportation to get me to the clinic, as if the problem with post-viral fatigue is losing the ability to google your local bus schedule. I spent months explaining how fatigue impacted me: I emailed, phoned consultants' secretaries, replied to letters that detailed every conversation. A year in, the only form of communication I hadn't tried was the medium of charades (two words: 'SHIT SHOW'). I hoped they were beginning to accept it. I hoped they were willing to give me the access arrangements I needed to get the treatment that was possible to receive at home. In fact, they referred me to social services. It turns out every remote appointment I had had over the last year had been logged as 'non-attendance'. Being too ill to leave the house was seen as 'non-compliance'.

The social worker was kind and helpful and I took it matter-of-factly as she spoke. My claim that I couldn't physically make it to appointments needed a 'safeguard check', I was told. I wondered, as a polite stranger asked for details about my body, how exactly we'd got here. I wondered whether a medic would refer a non-disabled person to social services after they had been in regular contact and showed no signs of distress, or suggest that they needed a social worker to help them make basic decisions about their healthcare. I wondered what exactly it took for medics to believe someone with a disability had authority and knowledge of their own health, or whether they would have been able to trust someone else who didn't happen to look like me. In the course of one phone call, every cultural prejudice about disabled women was exposed. That we are faking. Difficult. Too childlike to know our own minds. That this prejudice was coming from healthcare professionals meant to help me made it feel infinitely worse.

And yet I am white, slim, educated, and straight, and go into medical appointments with a heap of advantages. If you are a disabled woman of colour, LGBTQ+, live in poverty or are fat, you are at considerably more risk of experiencing poor care. Just as bias in healthcare affects the diagnosis marginalized disabled women receive, research overwhelmingly shows hidden biases fuel their inadequate treatment. Take the LGBTQ+ community. Research by the charity Stonewall in 2018[34] found almost a quarter of LGBTQ+ patients (23 per cent) had witnessed negative remarks about LGBTQ+ people from healthcare staff while accessing services. One in seven LGBTQ+ people (14 per cent) said they have avoided treatment altogether for fear of the discrimination they may face. Of those who do seek support, one in eight (13 per cent) have experienced some form of unequal treatment from healthcare staff because they're LGBTQ+. Transgender people with disabilities can be particularly vulnerable to discrimination in healthcare. According to the 2015 US Transgender Survey, 42 per cent of disabled respondents reported a negative experience when seeing a healthcare provider in the past year, compared to 30 per cent of transgender respondents without disabilities.[35]

Things are no easier for people of colour. A landmark study in 2022 found the majority of black people living in Britain have reported being discriminated against by healthcare professionals because of their race.[36] This bias starts young: the national survey found 75 per cent of black people aged between eighteen and thirty-four have experienced prejudice while visiting doctors and hospitals. Studies have long shown that black patients' pain is treated less seriously than their white counterparts. A 2012 meta-analysis[37] of twenty years of published research found that black patients were 22 per cent less likely than their white counterparts to get any pain medication, and 29 per cent less likely to be treated with opioids. A key explanation is the attitudes of healthcare workers and their in-built bias. One 2016 study[38] found half of the medical students surveyed held one or more racial prejudice about pain, including the false belief that black people's skin is thicker than white people's and the myth that black people's nerve endings are less sensitive. This has a clear knock-on effect on the treatment people of colour receive: the study showed trainees who believed that black people are not as sensitive to pain as white people were less likely to treat black people's pain appropriately.

Dr Emma Sheppard, a lecturer in Sociology at Aberystwyth University who has the chronic pain condition fibromyalgia herself, explains that disabled women who are also from other marginalized groups frequently have their disability 'blamed' on their minority status. 'Chronic conditions often become a part of what I call the "trans broken arm" problem – any medical issue is thought to be the result of the patient being trans, or fat, or a person of colour. This obscures the actual issue to the extent that it impacts the care they receive. Sometimes this can take the form of invasive and pointless questioning – for example, a trans person presenting with a broken arm being asked a lot of questions about surgery or HRT. Or for fat folks, this means that "diet and exercise" becomes the cure for everything. And when "exercise" is *already* a cure (as we know is falsely said to be the case for some health conditions, like ME or fibromyalgia), it becomes even more pressurized. This can be particularly an issue for women of colour with high BMIs. Assumptions get made about the person – that they're drug seeking, or involved in gang violence, or have poor diet – which can add to those issues of body size and, in turn, impact the treatment they receive.'

As Sheppard suggests, as well as race and gender identity, research has consistently shown that healthcare professionals are often biased against people deemed as being overweight. A study by University College London in 2022 found widespread 'weight stigma' across multiple countries and types of health staff.[39] Their analysis found that a number of healthcare professionals believe their patients of higher weight are 'lazy, lack self-control, overindulge, are hostile, dishonest, have poor hygiene and do not follow guidance'. Such prejudice was reported to have a deep effect on patients, leaving them stressed, anxious, and even skipping medical appointments. Tellingly, some fat patients reported that they were happier during the coronavirus pandemic lockdowns – when NHS services held online sessions for treatments – because they received less prejudice. No one could see them. This bias isn't just distressing – it's been found to have a direct impact on the quality of treatment fat women receive. When healthcare workers blame serious health issues on weight, they can inadvertently ignore other genuine causes. In one 2016 study,[40] 52 per cent of women said that their weight had been a barrier to receiving appropriate healthcare.

Journalist and author Ione Gamble, who has Crohn's disease and depression, has first-hand experience with this sort of prejudice from doctors. 'I was lucky – and skinnier – when

I was diagnosed with Crohn's, so my weight was never used as a detriment or held against me when seeking treatment. [As I gained weight] my weight has been an issue with the GP and other specialists when I'm seeking advice or treatment for new symptoms or other diagnoses I have, such as PCOS [polycystic ovary syndrome]. I've been told the only treatment for PCOS is weight loss and denied medication or further tests. I also think I was diagnosed with PCOS for my weight despite the fact that not all of my symptoms point to that as the cause of my uterus pain. With GPs, or in our medical system in general, the answer to all and any problems when you are fat is to lose weight, without any further investigation as to whether there is anything more serious or totally unrelated going on. I've even had experiences in which doctors have said my depression will be due to the fact I'm fat. I've been told my asthma is due to my weight. It's as though the first port of call is always weight despite the fact that there is no relation. It's something that fundamentally has to change as so many people are not being provided with adequate treatment.'

It takes a village

It's a strange beast to deal with, permanent illness. Humans are used to acute health problems – a chesty cough, a broken arm. The sort that can be fixed, patched up and healed. We are not designed for lasting sickness, the sort that rears its head on an ordinary Thursday morning and is still there years later, like an unwelcome house guest. When

I became chronically ill, I had no idea how to tread this new terrain. Diagnosis and treatment by healthcare teams was certainly lacking, but more than that, there seemed to be next to no access to care and support networks. When medics were unable to fix my symptoms, I craved information about how to live with them. Much more, I craved to know how to live *well* with them. How could I pace my limited energy to get things done? When my pain is spiking, what do I do? If I look three months pregnant from codeine bloating, what should I name the baby?* Or to put it another way: how do you live when 'recovery' never comes? If the TV stops working, you can turn to the instruction manual. And yet when it's your body, too often you're expected to figure it out alone.

When journalist Natasha Lipman was diagnosed with Ehlers–Danlos syndrome aged twenty-one after years of health problems, she began to feel hopeful she could get advice on how to live with the condition. But in reality, she found that having a name to put to her symptoms was not enough to 'unlock the door' to support. 'Despite having access to good-quality healthcare, there wasn't any advice [from medics] on how to live with my condition. I remember being told by a pain management psychologist to "expect less" of my life. It felt like I was being treated like a collection of individual body parts, not a person with hopes and dreams and a whole life ahead of me. In the

* Co-co.

170

end, I just gave up on everything as my body declined and I became more and more housebound.

'I was directed to online forums for peer support but they were overwhelmingly negative, an environment where older people were telling younger people like me about how bad their lives were going to become. I understand it now – many of them were struggling without care and support for decades – but it was terrifying. It was the first time I felt scared about the future. It's a shame because there are some really wonderful spaces online. What I really needed was support to properly understand my condition and all the different ways to "manage" it, taking into consideration what was important to me in my life.'

Faced with a lack of diversity and understanding in formal healthcare settings, the disabled community have created networks to support themselves and others to navigate life with a long-term health condition. Chronic Illness Inclusion[41] – a group specifically for people with fatigue or pain – provides advice and lobbying for practical aspects of health problems, including access to benefits, employment, and ableism in healthcare. WinVisible[42] – a community group for disabled women, which works to be inclusive of immigrants, refugees, and women with invisible disabilities – provides information and advocacy on areas ranging from healthcare, employment, to transport. Elsewhere, 'But You Don't Look Sick'[43] provides an online community that connects people with different chronic conditions.

Lipman herself went on to create The Rest Room, a podcast that aims to help people live well with chronic conditions, and stresses several practical tips for how to manage our health. 'Take time to understand your body. This might sound silly – of course most of us with long-term health problems spend a huge amount of time thinking about our bodies and feeling acutely aware of them. But actually learning to notice and understand our bodies is a different thing. For example, I have fatigue and a big part of learning to understand when I'm pushing myself too far has been to check in with what my body does when I start doing that. So for me, when I start feeling my heart beat faster or I get warm, it's a sign that I've started pushing myself too far. Recognizing and paying attention to them means that I can in theory stop before I crash.

'Secondly, if you're looking to make progress, start slow. Slower than you think. If you struggle to read, start with a single sentence. If you are going out for dinner soon but are always in your pyjamas, perhaps start by having a "day pyjama" top you change into every day to ease yourself in to the exertion of getting ready. The aim is always to do things that are safe and sustainable for where your body is right now. Where we often end up getting in trouble is that we are pushed to do too much too quickly. It's [also] useful to find people who are going through what you are. Luckily, great online support groups do exist now, as well as social media accounts. As physiotherapist Jackie Walumbe told me when I interviewed her for my podcast: "When they say it takes a village to raise a child, I think it takes a village to live with a chronic illness because you build your village around you.'"

That village can include this sort of support for how to physically manage our health condition, but it can also mean finding help with how to cope with it emotionally. Long-term physical health problems naturally take a toll on our mental health, whether that's anxiety about symptoms, shame about the things we can't do, or depression from isolation. I know during the course of my illness I have felt helpless, frustrated, and scared. Carrying all that emotional baggage is tough at the best of times but I already had very weak arms. On top of this, disabled women's mental health can be affected by the inequality we face. Tropes around disability ('poor you!') mean it's often assumed any sadness or anger we feel is because of our bodies, but how society discriminates against us can cause significantly more damage. Living day-to-day with ableism on top of sexism (and any other prejudice minorities may face) can be hugely stressful – and is proven to take a serious toll on our wellbeing. A 2022 report by the World Health Organization into the health inequalities of disabled people[44] found those with severe disabilities have a 2.5-fold higher likelihood of having depression. Other studies have suggested that disabled people are up to three times more likely to experience depression than non-disabled people, as well as being at more risk of anxiety.[45]

While disabled women can suffer particular strains on our mental health, it's often harder for us to access professional help. NHS mental health waiting times mean many patients are forced to wait months or years for an appointment or to pay to go private, meaning disabled people – who are more likely to be on a low income than other groups[46] –can find ourselves priced out of support. At the same time, the counselling room can come with physical barriers, from worksheets that aren't accessible for visually impaired patients, language obstacles for hearing-impaired people who use British Sign Language, to therapists not wearing masks to protect clients who are immunocompromised. For all its strengths, the NHS can unfortunately be particularly inflexible to disabled people seeking mental health support: many services require in-person sessions and don't allow remote access, while if our health means we have to skip appointments, we may be considered 'not committed' and discharged from the list.

If you're struggling with your mental health – and it's OK if you are – it can be useful to talk to your GP who can explore options like the possibility of medication, such as antidepressants and anxiety medicine, if that's right for you. They can discuss with you what therapeutic services are available on the NHS locally, while it's also possible to self-refer to some services that may have shorter waiting times. Don't be afraid to be open about your access needs from the off and to talk them through with your GP or private provider.* It's a big enough leap to ask for help; you should never have to worry about whether you're able to take it.

In recent years, 'self-care' has become a buzzword on social media, denoting anything from buying an over-priced candle to going for a run and then taking a selfie of that run (#endorphins #womenwhorun #bestlife). And yet many of the techniques that dominate the media can feel alien to women with disabilities. Having a healthy woman named Arabella urge me to go wild swimming for my mental health is not much use when I'm struggling to get out of bed. This can be all the harder if you used to be able to do physical exercise; instead of going for a run making you feel better, you end up feeling worse about the fact you can't go for a run any more (helpful). On top of that, women with disabilities and health conditions are often going through things that many others aren't, which means mainstream care tips can feel inadequate. Magazines and influencers might tell us how to self-care our way around a bad break-up or annoying colleague but, funnily enough, rarely cover how to cope with a pain flare or stressful hospital appointment. On the other hand, young

---

* If you're struggling to access mental health services that suit your dis-ability, take another look at the tips at the start of this chapter about how to get the most from medical appointments.

women struggling with their health can be vulnerable to the exploitative side of the 'wellness' trend, where online accounts promise that some kale, positive thinking, and extortionately priced supplements will cure us of illness or disability. Share concerns about your health on social media and you'll likely either get spam offering the number for an 'alternative' doctor's office or a stranger replying that they'll pray for the love of Jesus Christ to heal you. As disabled women, finding ways to nurture ourselves in the face of all this that work for both our unique bodies and circumstances can be invaluable.

Anna HeardinLondon, a confidence coach who herself has hypermobility, endometriosis and long Covid, has adapted traditional self-care advice to make it work for those of us with disabilities. 'Tips like "get moving" can initially look like something that only people who have average bodies can do but we get to make our own rules. What movement feels joyful to you? Is it a kitchen disco? Is it covering your hands in paint and seeing which weird ways your wrists move on paper? What idea of moving makes you smile and giggle at how ridiculous it sounds? Do more of that. And if you want, involve people you love and who love you.

'Or get out into nature, however that is possible for you. Maybe it's making the effort to watch a sunset or to open a window and feel the rain in your face. If you're unable to leave the house, is there a plant that you could investigate as if it's the first time you have ever met? Which is the smell, the texture, the curve of the leaf? How gentle can you be with the soil? Spend some time with it. What haven't you noticed before? Could you fill a bowl with water? Dip just your toes in and spend some time remembering the best beach you have ever visited, in great detail. Yes, getting outside is wonderful. But when we can't get there, do not miss how vast inside can be too.'

'It's absolutely OK to ask for help, rest, feel overwhelmed, take your time, make mistakes, feel all the emotions,' stresses psychotherapist and NHS consultant therapist Nikki Jack, who herself has atypical cystic fibrosis, chronic pain and fatigue. 'Sometimes, we're struggling more than we admit. We say "I'm fine" when we aren't. Maybe you are too exhausted to explain, scared you will get emotional if you say how you really feel, or worried you'll sound as though you're complaining, exaggerating or a burden.

'I've been there too, putting on a brave face and hiding how I really feel, sometimes from myself! One of the most important things I've learned, and also share with others, is that struggling doesn't mean we're failing or a burden. The more we can open up and talk about our feelings, the easier it is to understand them. Next time someone asks, "How are you?" consider something like, "I want to say 'I'm fine' but I'm not" or "There is a lot happening, do you have time to listen?" No one tells us how lonely chronic illness and disability can feel. If you feel very isolated and alone, or no one asks how you're doing any more, please speak to

a professional or trusted person and ask them for help to
find the right support for you.'

If you're a non-disabled person reading this who loves
someone with a chronic illness or disability, it's natural to
not always know how to be that 'trusted person'. Illness is a
bit like miscarriage or death – many of us don't really know
how to talk about it. The truth is, there are no magic words
to say to support someone struggling with their health. Just
showing up – and keeping showing up – will be of help,
whether that's asking them how they're feeling or distract-
ing them from a bad day with filthy gossip. Simply checking
in with a 'How have you been?' WhatsApp message is a
good start, even if you've been quiet for a while. You might
want to also offer practical support, from driving them back
from a hospital appointment to bringing them shopping
while they're in a flare-up. (And don't be offended if they
say, 'No thanks.') Whatever you do, at its core, it will say
something important: that this thing that is happening to
them is real, and that you care.

In many ways, this book is dedicated to dispelling the
myth that having a health condition means you can't
have a great, fulfilling life. That's important. But I'm also
never going to pretend it can't be hard sometimes; really
hard. Not for every condition. Not for every person. And
certainly not all the time. But still, hard. Acknowledging

that health problems are tough – and giving ourselves permission to feel that way – seems like it should be the most natural thing, but the narratives around sickness mean we're often sent the message that this is wrong. When we talk about health, there is typically a push to be 'strong' and 'brave'. Newspapers describe famous cancer patients as facing 'a battle'. Social media praises chronically ill people as being 'warriors'. Established wisdom says the best medicine for ill health is positivity: 'Chin up!' Much of this language can be well-meaning – a clumsy attempt to elevate a community of people who are too often perceived as weak or to 'chivvy along' an upset friend – but this narrative is not ultimately helpful. It perpetuates the false idea that 'the only disability is a bad mental attitude', as if a paraplegic's legs would rise up if only they smiled more. It also encourages people with health conditions to embrace toxic positivity – that is, the idea that we should try to only feel or show positive traits – which manages to both invalidate what we are going through and force us to ignore what we are actually feeling. It is essentially the health equivalent of someone saying they've just lost all their worldly possessions in a fire, and then being asked why they look so sad. This pressure is all the more if you're a woman, with 'the fairer sex' still socialized to be cheerful ('Smile, love!') and all things nice. Strong negative emotions – fear, anger, anxiety – are a natural response to health problems (hell, it's a natural response to life), and we shouldn't have to repress them when they come up. What's more, experts agree it's better for us if we don't.

There's a reason we reach for an Adele album when we're heartbroken.

Dr Sula Windgassen, a health psychologist who previously had bladder pain syndrome herself, explains. 'People often worry that they will wallow or downward-spiral if they acknowledge a difficult emotional experience. The result is that they often suppress or push away emotions, but that's not a long-term strategy. Acknowledging emotions can be as simple as checking in with how you're feeling once a day and asking yourself what you need. Make this a regular habit to help honour your own needs and acknowledge your own worth.

'[If you find yourself worrying,] try to identify what specifically it is you're worrying about in a given moment and to categorize this worry. Is this something that hasn't yet happened that may not happen? In which case it is out of your control. Is this something that has happened but you can't do anything about it? In which case this is also out of your control. Or is this something that is happening or about to happen that you do have a degree of control over? In this case, focus on the degree of control, make a plan and enact that plan or schedule it in. One of the most powerful practices you can learn is to let go – whether that's from sticky thought streams, plans that can no longer happen because of your health, or expectations that may not be fulfilled. To let go of what you can't control is to find peace.'

Anna HeardinLondon says writing things down – rather than just thinking them – can be another useful tool. 'When things seem hard or confusing, I always find it helpful to get it out of my head and on to paper. You don't even need to know what you want to write, but just get a pen on a piece of paper and fill it with everything that flows into your brain as it pops up. From this list of stuff you have just poured on to paper, try and sift through it and work out what is a fact and what is a story you have been telling yourself. For example, if I'm having a slow day and my body isn't responding, I might "brain dump" things like "I should be able to do more today" or "It doesn't matter if I overdo it, I never feel well anyway." I like to imagine myself picking these thoughts up with tweezers and examining them from all angles and, without judgement, asking: is this thought serving me? If I decide it is not, rather than trying to toxic-positivity my way out of it, I try to neutralize it by practising thoughts like "this is a human body" or "these are human legs". It strips things back to the facts rather than the drama.

'On top of this, I think one of the best investments you can make for yourself is an "In case of emergency" box – a little treasure trove of self-care you can dip into when you need. Fill it with lyrics which have moved you, colours which calm you, photos which make your heart light up, love letters to yourself, smells which bring back memories. Write down your victories in your own words, actively celebrate your wins, especially your tiny ones. The more you build your own toolkit, the better. Slowly, you will begin to train your brain to remember you are someone who can survive hard stuff and that you have the resources inside yourself.'

It is easy to chastise your body for 'failing', but as Anna HeardinLondon recommends, I try to feel pride in its victories instead. Mine copes with more most days than other people's do in a decade, and I'm guessing yours might do too. If you're struggling to feel pride in yourself right now, or just struggling generally, it doesn't mean that's how it will always be. Just like there is often no end point to chronic illness or disability, there is no end point for learning how to cope with it either. There is no perfect epiphany where everything suddenly falls into place, no finish line that with enough training or effort we can somehow cross. Chronic health conditions are less a marathon to complete and more one of those corporate team-building exercises where you wander around a forest blindfolded: a hell of a lot of work and you don't necessarily feel like you're getting anywhere. Here's the good news: you are. Every day you wake up and try again is a day when you are moving. Every day you take your meds and drink some water is a day you are showing up and caring for yourself. Progress is not linear. Your ability to cope is not static or fixed in stone. There will be days when it seems like you've got a handle on things. There will be days when you wonder whether a four-finger KitKat counts as breakfast (it does). A wobble does not undo the gains you've been making, just like how you feel today does not define how you will feel tomorrow. You're finding it hard because it *is* hard. And you're carrying on regardless.

This might be a good time to say I'm proud of you. I just wanted to tell you in case no one has lately.

All tits and teeth

One morning in my early twenties, my teeth started to throb. The rest of this anecdote should be dull but straightforward: I booked an appointment with my dentist and I felt better. Except, I didn't have one. In fact, I hadn't seen a dentist since I was a teenager. As a wheelchair user, the dental surgery that the rest of my family had long used was inaccessible to me. Dental practices in the UK are not dissimilar to your schoolfriend's older brother who sells weed: highly sought-after but often run out of the top floor of the local barber's. Without being on any dentist's books and with no idea how to quickly find an accessible surgery, I did what people in pain do: queued for hours in a dental walk-in centre located on an industrial estate. In the end, a dentist fixed my problem (plot twist: I was grinding my teeth), but it left me all too aware of a bigger one: I had struggled to access a basic form of healthcare, just because I had a disability.

We've seen in this chapter that it can be difficult to get a diagnosis or treatment for your long-term health condition.

But if you're disabled, it isn't just hard to get healthcare for your disability – it can be hard to access healthcare completely unrelated to it. The regular health checks that most women rightly take for granted are often blocked off from those of us with disabilities. This happens at the most basic level – like being able to see your own primary-care doctor. A YouGov survey commissioned by Leonard Cheshire in 2020[47] found nearly a quarter (24 per cent) of disabled adults have experienced problems accessing key services where they live, including GP surgeries.

Broadcaster Samantha Renke, who is three feet nine inches tall due to a brittle bone condition, knows what it's like to be unable to access a basic health service. 'I still can't find an accessible GP practice. They're either not in walking distance from my home – I struggle to use public transport because of my disability – or have a private car park but don't have a sufficient kerb for a safe exit from a taxi with a wheelchair. Even having to pay for a taxi to get there is a barrier, just another extra disability cost. If I can get inside, it's not much better. There are the high reception desks, all those little computer iPads that you need to sign yourself in with which are often out of reach to me. I've had a number of rather ableist and ignorant receptionists who have absolutely dismissed me when I tried to talk to them. They speak to my PA instead.'

Being able to access the same primary-care doctor has been vital for Sarah Gordy MBE over the years. As a woman with Down's syndrome, the actor is highly aware of the unequal healthcare many learning disabled people face. 'I'm lucky to have had the same GP for a long time. I also have family who support me. I was very upset when I visited an old friend from school with Down's syndrome. After her parents died, she lived in a flat run by the council and had support workers. She was diabetic. I saw on the fridge the care workers had a list of her meals and they were not healthy, completely wrong for a diabetic. She got bigger and bigger. That made it harder to move around and she got out of breath. I tried to support her with her diet but was away a lot with work. I was very sad when she died. It was too soon. I know people with learning disabilities can have a hard time with healthcare. I worked with [the learning disability charity] Mencap on a film for their Get It Right campaign where my character was in pain and wasn't getting the help she needed. I also acted in a General Medical Council training film to help doctors learn about treating patients like me. Doctors and nurses need to have the time to talk to patients and understand them. And people like me need extra time for that.'

As Gordy and Renke know, ableist attitudes in healthcare aren't just frustrating – they can be a barrier to disabled women and non-binary people getting the medical support we need. Perhaps few areas show this more than reproductive care. Cultural beliefs around disability and sex mean that many non-disabled people still believe myths such as disabled women don't have sexual relationships or can't or shouldn't become a mum – a prejudice that healthcare workers are not immune from. Research shows this sort of bias has a knock-on effect on whether we receive the same access to sex-based services other women do. A two-year study by the charity Engender in 2018[48] found disabled women in Scotland face significant barriers to reproductive healthcare. The research described how failures in reproductive, sexual and maternal health services see healthcare workers infantilize their disabled patients, as well as make negative or stereotyped assumptions about them. In extreme cases, this poor treatment led to disabled women having forced abortions or sterilizations and even the unfounded removal of their children into care.

As a blind mum-to-be, disability consultant Dr Amy Kavanagh faced discrimination frequently by some of her maternal healthcare team when pregnant with her first child. 'I was horrified by how unprepared the staff at the leading maternity hospital in London were for a blind or disabled parent. I wanted a water birth – and ended up having a beautiful one – but I was initially refused permission to use the birthing pool on the basis that I would have to "step in and out" and that they would need eight people to lift me out of the pool. The antenatal team couldn't comprehend that my blindness didn't affect my mobility. I asked if they were so concerned, why couldn't they use a hoist. They replied that they didn't have a hoist on the labour ward. When I asked what would happen if a wheelchair-using parent needed to use a hoist to be examined, I was met with stony silence.

'The worst incident was during my gestational diabetes test, where you drink a very sugary liquid to test your blood sugar levels. My partner accompanied me to the hospital as usual but when we were called into the clinical room the nurse refused to let him in. We tried to insist that he was my named carer in my notes but they wouldn't budge. Then the nurse tried to make my partner take my guide dog Ava out of the room. We refused, stating she was my eyes and supporting me. The nurse proceeded to shout at me and become very abusive. She was furious when I repeatedly explained I couldn't read the small print on the forms during the test and that she'd removed the person who could read things for me. When I was trying to finish the disgusting sugary drink, she grabbed the packet. Then she shoved the drink in my mouth and forced the liquid down my throat. It was incredibly traumatic and dehumanizing. The nurse was angry at me for being blind and decided to physically punish me because I wouldn't comply in the way she wanted. The hospital were so anxious about me escalating the incident into a serious complaint they rolled out the red carpet afterwards.'

This sort of discrimination is shocking but far from the only dire consequence of unequal healthcare. Disabled women are frequently blocked from accessing potentially life-saving care, at risk to our lives. A smear test – a preventative procedure that can help show up early signs of cervical cancer – on the NHS is available to anyone with a cervix over the age of twenty-five. It's common for the media to report that nerves mean young women are sometimes reluctant to attend a smear test, but if you're disabled you may struggle to even get the chance to go. A survey by Jo's Cervical Cancer Trust in 2019 found that 63 per cent of women with physical disabilities had been unable to attend a screening due to their disability.[49] Almost half said they had chosen not to attend a smear in the past due to a previous bad experience or fears about how health professionals might react. According to the most recent figures available, only 34 per cent of women with a learning disability eligible for cervical cancer screenings received a smear test, compared to 75 per cent of eligible non-disabled women.[50]

Zoe Lloyd, campaign manager at the charity Enhance UK which runs the Undressing Disability campaign, and who herself has rheumatoid arthritis, says there are multiple reasons for this. 'Doctors can often make the assumption that a disabled person isn't sexually active so they aren't offered a screening. Or there are practical problems, such as once you get to the appointment, you find the bed isn't adjustable for you to get on to and the clinic doesn't have a hoist. There might also be poor accessibility in public health messaging, such as radio adverts excluding Deaf clients or television ads not being captioned. This can also be the case for sexually transmitted disease checks. When our charity did a giveaway of STI kits, three hundred kits went in three weeks, showing there's a huge need for home tests.'

When Renke had her first cervical screening in rural Lancashire aged twenty-five, the procedure went smoothly. But since she moved to London ten years ago, every smear test has been 'a nightmare'. 'I guess no one really likes going for a smear test and having a stranger fiddling around with your private parts. But for me and many disabled people, having an awkward medical examination is the least of my problems. I've had GPs in the past be rather uncomfortable that someone with a disability is sexually active and seeking sexual health advice. We're so often infantilized. Then there's the logistical problems. None of the GPs that I go to have a hoist so I need someone to help me on to the examination bed. Most of the beds don't go low enough to meet a safe transfer and not all my PAs are strong enough to lift me. At times, I've struggled to get a care support package and had to rely on friends to assist me but a smear is not something I particularly want to ask them to help me with.

'As I have a petite frame, it's no shock that my vagina is also petite. This means that most GPs and even hospitals I've visited to get a smear test or a colposcopy haven't got the correct speculums. I literally feel like Goldilocks and the three speculums when I go for a smear test. "This one's too big, this one's too small . . ." Because the equipment isn't correct, I'm often prodded and probed for an unhealthy and uncomfortable amount of time. On one occasion, I was asked to jump on to a birthing chair with stirrups. As someone who has non-union fractures in both of her legs and her legs are incredibly short, this was a ludicrous suggestion. It all makes a simple routine procedure rather traumatic.'

Just like with smear tests, disabled women are significantly less likely than non-disabled women to opt for a mammogram when invited for one. Women in the UK are eligible for a breast screening on the NHS from the age of fifty,[51] while any-aged woman can be referred by their GP if, for example, they find a lump or other symptom. Spotting the early signs of cancer are crucial as the sooner it is found and treated, the better the chances of recovery. But research by the University of Oxford and funded by Cancer Research UK found that disabled women are a third less likely to participate in screenings for breast cancer than non-disabled women.[52] The same study showed women with disabilities were also a quarter less likely than their non-disabled peers to have a bowel cancer screening. This is not a case of women simply deciding not to go to their appointments, rather they often don't have a genuine choice to attend. Researchers found disabled women miss out on cancer screenings due to many access reasons, from a lack of accessible transport to get to the clinic to the fact that wheelchair users often can't reach the traditional mammogram machines from their chairs. Unsurprisingly, the more affected a woman is by health conditions, the harder it is for her to access healthcare: the study found women with two or more disabilities were less likely to take part in cancer screenings compared to women who had just one disability.

Whether it's a smear test, sexual health check, or just a dentist's appointment, disabled women deserve the same access to safe and dignified healthcare as our non-disabled peers – and we can turn to each other for advice on how to get it. For Trishna Bharadia, health advocate and a visiting lecturer in patient engagement at King's College London, who herself has MS, the key to a successful medical appointment is being prepared. 'I always say don't be shy in being upfront about what your requirements are. Don't assume that someone will know about your disability or your condition. Preparation is key and contacting the healthcare team prior to the appointment can be really beneficial. If it's the first time you're going for a particular test, then ask the team to describe in detail what it will involve so that you can identify as far as possible any issues that might arise. If you've had the test before, then share with the team what worked and didn't work and explain that you're speaking from experience. Be open and honest, but also firm about what you need. If possible, ask for a longer appointment time – and explain why – so that if things do take longer or issues arise at the time, there's no sense of having to rush in order to get the test done so that the next patient can be seen. The bookings clerk may not be able to do this so it's worth speaking to your GP or the secretary of the consultant who has ordered the test for them to arrange this.'

When it comes to sexual health checks, this might mean going to a specialist clinic rather than a standard hospital. Dr Helen Dring-Turner, who leads neuro-divergence work at Brook, a nationwide sexual health charity, and herself has a chronic respiratory and auto-immune condition, says there are many ways to access clinic services for disabled clients. 'If you're worried about having an STI or an unwanted pregnancy, Brook has a Find a Service tool on our website[*] where you can find a Brook clinic or another local sexual health service. Brook's clinics are open to all, and we provide a range of additional support for disabled people including hearing induction loop systems, chaperones and interpreters, and informa-tion in easy-read format. We also have step-free access and accessible toilets at our clinics as standard. You can find details of the specific support available at each of our clinics through the Find a Service tool. Sometimes there are specific specialist services for disabled people – for example, The Bridge which supports those with learning disabilities or autism. If there's not, it's best to call ahead (or get a carer or friend to call ahead) to understand the clinic's accessibility and whether they have experience with your condition.

* brook.org.uk/find-a-service

'If you need someone to go to a sexual health clinic with you for support, the clinic will usually like to see you on your own first. If you don't understand anything at your appointment, please ask the nurse or wellbeing worker to explain again. The nurse will take the time to help you understand. If you struggle to physically access a clinic, don't worry – many sexual health services can now be accessed digitally. For example, STI tests can be ordered online and be delivered to your home.'

Fleur Perry, a former volunteer for the patients-rights charity Healthwatch, who uses a wheelchair and BiPAP due to spinal muscular atrophy, has had many medical appointments over the years 'where things have not gone right' and has developed tools to get better care. 'I've booked a hoist and then been told to stand by an X-ray screen. I've had a physio almost dislocate my shoulder because she didn't stop when I was in pain. I've been overdosed, ignored, and prodded. I've learned, firstly, give yourself time. If you know that you're not being treated correctly, say something to create that time, like "Please stop" or "I'm going to take a break." In a long appointment, don't ask for a break, tell them you are taking a break. Practise saying these phrases at home beforehand if you need. Once you're calm, state the facts as they are, and say what needs to happen. Try "That's not safe for me. We need to do this a different way" or "I disagree. That doesn't match my experience. Tell me more options please."

'If they don't make things work for you and can't give a proper reason why, please don't take that first answer. Ask to see someone else – if a medical professional has lost your trust, you can ask for a second opinion. Your health and your needs are important, and only you know what is best for you. It can be difficult complaining if something bad happens. You might feel like they won't listen anyway, or they might be more unfriendly next time. Pick your battles to conserve your energy, but every time you are listened to will pave the way for others to be heard. That's priceless. And you deserve that.'

As this chapter has shown, women with disabilities and chronic conditions are up against many inequalities in the healthcare system: from the biases held by some healthcare professionals towards disabled people and other marginalized groups, inaccessible wider medical services, to the need for more help to live well with our symptoms. And yet we have also seen that there are strategies we can use to advocate for ourselves, and that the disabled community are at the forefront of providing support for each other as we fight for change. Maybe you're struggling to get healthcare right now. Maybe your own curtains are on fire. I'm not going to insult you by saying everything is going to be magically OK, as if platitudes will fix prejudice or your symptoms will ease with the right words. But I will say this: you deserve to be believed by every medic you meet. You deserve to receive the same quality of treatment as anyone else. You deserve fully rounded psychological and practical support from a system that sees your quality of life as valuable. Oh and a complimentary dachshund trained to collect your meds from the pharmacy via a tiny trailer he pulls by his tail. Change in the healthcare system may be slow. It may be disheartening or outright infuriating. But we are getting there, bit by bit, together, like we always do. (Free dachshunds might take longer to achieve, though, I won't lie.)

Relationships

'I never knew whether I should disclose my disability when I was talking to somebody [on a dating app]. I never wanted to blurt it out as the first thing, "HELLO I AM DISABLED", but then, if I didn't tell them at the beginning, I got worried that they would accuse me of catfishing.'

— Rosie Jones

When I was eighteen, strangers would carry me up stairs. After moving from a small town to a city for university, I had the luck of being near one of the greatest clubs in the country for gigs. For the next ten years, I loved going there with friends; the smell of smoke and ticket stubs lining the floor. And yet being one of the 'greatest' clubs in the UK did not mean being accessible. Without a single lift or ramp, the only way into the main hall was up two flights of stairs. The alternative was a fire exit up (there will be no prizes for guessing) . . . a flight of stairs. To get inside, four bouncers had to hoist me aloft in my wheelchair, like a pharaoh on wheels. For anyone who has never been lifted into a building by four men, this is not as erotic as it sounds. One man is invariably pressed to your chest, two others grappling at your legs, but not in a sexy way. More a fear-of-brain-injury way. The price of a night out with friends was more than the £15 door price – it was basic safety. And yet I did it. I did it unthinkingly, over and over for years. I wanted a social life like everyone else – and sometimes that meant holding on to the arm of a man named Big Steve and contemplating my own mortality.

If you'd have asked me when I was growing up whether my disability was relevant to my friendships or dates, I'd have said 'no' – and probably been offended that you'd asked. Disability is one of those things I didn't give enough credit to in my twenties, like drinking water regularly. But it has always been there, sewn through the lively nights out and the lonely nights in. Being carried into my friends' twenty-first birthday party because the cocktail bar had multiple types of vodka but no lift. The man who asked me out online but ghosted me when I mentioned I used a wheelchair. The unrivalled happiness of sitting in a pub with friends again after being too fatigued to see them for months. Whether it's societal attitudes, physical access or my own body, at some point my disability has impacted every type of relationship in my life.

In some ways, it feels strange to write a chapter about this. Spending time with friends, having sex or falling in love are such basic parts of being human that they shouldn't warrant much attention. But that these things are entirely ordinary is surely the point. Disabled women grow up in a world where we are told that what everyone else has 'is not for people like you', where everyday experiences like orgasms, drinks with friends or becoming a mum are still taboo if your body happens to be different. From the myth that disabled women can't have romantic partners, the epidemic of disabled loneliness, to the erasure of disabled sexual pleasure, women and non-binary people with disabilities and health conditions still face multiple hurdles to enjoy the relationships non-disabled people expect. But that doesn't mean we aren't having them – one bouncer lift at a time.

Undateable

There are some myths in life that refuse to die. Don't go for a swim after a big meal. Dogs can't look up. Disabled people don't have relationships. I can't speak for the evidence of all of them (presumably someone had a bad experience eating spaghetti at a lido) but I will weigh in on that last one. To put it bluntly, many non-disabled people are still weirded out about the idea that disabled women date, enjoy sex or have kids.

Research in the journal *Human Sexuality*[1] in 2022 found myths around intimate relationships and disability to be prevalent in society, including the idea people with disabilities have no sexual desires or interests, that non-disabled people would not find someone with a disability desirable, and that it's easier for someone with a disability to adapt to sexual losses and change. One interesting study[2] had a focus group of disabled and non-disabled people view a documentary about sex and disability. It found that across the board disabled people were predominantly viewed as asexual and that there was a stigma attached to the idea of disabled people being sexual like non-disabled people.

This isn't just in focus groups – it's real life. Staggeringly, just 5 per cent of people in the UK who aren't disabled have ever asked out, or been on a date with, a disabled person, according to research by Scope.[3] A separate survey by Scope in 2022 into the impact prejudice around disability has on disabled people's lives found intimate relationships to be a key casualty: 77 per cent of disabled people who'd experienced negative attitudes said it had affected their romantic life, either by making dating less enjoyable, dating less than they would like to, or avoiding dates altogether.[4] This isn't just a case of the general public not looking to date a disabled person – there's evidence to suggest a partner becoming disabled leads some non-disabled people to end a relationship they're already in. Notably, that may be especially true for men. One study from the US found women are six times more likely to be left by their husband or boyfriend if they're diagnosed with cancer or multiple sclerosis than if their male partners were facing the same condition.[5]

Dr Kirsty Liddiard, senior research fellow in the School of Education and iHuman at the University of Sheffield, who has a neuromuscular disability, says: 'Disabled women are surrounded by cultural myths that say we are distinctly unwanted, unsexy and unattractive. Women's worth generally is judged by their bodies and attractiveness and their ability to both desire others and be desired. Yet for disabled women, there's a further layer of pressure – the assumption that because, for many of us, our bodies and minds may differ from the norm, we are relegated to being undesirable. Instead, disabled women's sexualities are largely understood in troubling ways. For example, some disabled women are assumed to lack the "capacity" to be able to understand sex, love and intimacy. Others are assumed to just not be interested – that we are sexless and that we don't have or want intimate relationships with others. And for some disabled women it's assumed sex is not physically possible.

'Part of this is about structural problems. Shitty accessibility and unemployment or underemployment mean disabled people still remain relatively excluded from the spaces we might meet partners, like pubs, clubs, work, and for some, online. And I think part of this comes from common misconceptions that exist around disabled people's lives. Ideas like disability is inherently tragic, that disabled people are *only* objects of care (or that caring for someone is inherently a negative experience) or that being disabled is something that makes you a poor girlfriend, husband or lover. We seldom get the chance to see or understand disability or disabled people as vibrant, sexy, fun, and as brilliant partners, parents and mates.'

It's not hard to see where these attitudes may come from. As Liddiard says, popular culture rarely depicts disabled women in happy, healthy relationships – or a relationship at all. I can count on one hand the number of times I've seen a disabled character on TV, film or in a novel dating like any other. The few times I have seen disabled people depicted in fictional relationships, it's largely negative, unhealthy or outright offensive. Think of *Me Before You*, the book-turned-film where a tetraplegic chooses to die by assisted suicide in order to give his caregiver and girlfriend the chance to live a full life without him. Reality shows are not much better. *Love Island*, arguably the biggest dating show of a generation, went years without having a disabled contestant; it took until 2022 for Tasha Ghouri, who uses a cochlear implant, to become the first woman with a disability to be chosen by producers.[6,7] Previously, ITV bosses had said the famous villa set isn't adapted for people with disabilities due to insurance costs and 'budget constraints'.[8] Instead, *The Undateables* – a show where disabled people are set up with a love interest based on the premise they are 'undateable' – has dominated the screen, a concept critics have called 'offensive' and 'exploitative'.[9] Even real-life campaigns around relationships and consent often fail to include disabled women. The #MeToo movement of the late 2010s was widely criticized by disabled activists[10] for inadvertently reinforcing stereotypes that women with disabilities[11] do not need to be concerned about unwanted attention. If disabled women aren't seen as attractive, why should they worry about men groping them?

In the few times disabled women are portrayed in culture as a wife, girlfriend or mother, it's often viewed as shocking by sections of the general public. When a sculpture of Alison Lapper – whose disability means she has no arms and shortened legs – was unveiled on the fourth plinth in Trafalgar Square in 2005, she received a barrage of negative comments. Some people called the 3.5-metre statue by Marc Quinn 'vulgar' and 'disgusting', with one aspect causing particular offence: she was depicted as heavily pregnant. As Lapper put it to the BBC in 2024, people thought 'she shouldn't be naked and pregnant and disabled and a single parent'.[12]

These myths have consequences. As we saw in the previous chapter, the belief that disabled women don't have intimate relationships contributes to the fact we often miss out on accessing gender-based services, from smear tests to accessible antenatal support. At the same time, women who are at risk in their relationships are frequently left without help: disabled women are twice as likely to be victims of domestic abuse by their partners than non-disabled women[13] but just one in ten refuges in the UK are accessible to people with physical disabilities.[14] Even the social security system assumes disabled people are perpetually single. Under current rules,[15] some people on disability benefits risk losing part, or all, of their financial support if they move in with a partner. That's not to mention the micro-aggressions about our sexuality that disabled women face day-to-day, from GPs thinking we don't need contraception to strangers assuming our boyfriend is our carer.

When Paralympic champion and peer Baroness Tanni Grey-Thompson became a mum, she found herself exposed to such prejudice. Over the years, Grey-Thompson, who uses a wheelchair due to spina bifida, has been repeatedly accosted by members of the public who didn't believe her daughter was hers. 'When I was about eight months pregnant, someone stopped me in the street and asked "Was I pregnant?" I genuinely didn't know what to say. They asked me how I got pregnant and they poked me, so I said, "I had sex with my husband." She was horrified. I was told that people like me shouldn't be allowed to have children. My answer to the "people like you" is always, "What do you mean, Welsh people?"'

'I was on a flight once when my daughter was about three years old. One of the airline crew got very agitated even though I was sitting next to her on the plane and they started saying, "There's a baby on-board, who brought the baby?" I can't remember exactly what happened next but there was a conversation about me not being a responsible adult and that I couldn't travel with her. A businessman who by then was sitting on the other side of us said that he would be the responsible adult for my daughter. The crew then seemed to be OK with that.'

For social entrepreneur and broadcaster Shani Dhanda, who has brittle bone disease, it was her own family who assumed her disability would rule her out of having a relationship. 'Growing up, my family never spoke to me about getting married. As a South Asian woman, where marriage is intrinsic to my culture, this is completely unheard of. On the one hand, I was relieved because I didn't want an arranged or introduced marriage. On the other, I was annoyed at being left out. As a young person born with a disability, I always wondered if I'd ever be in a relationship or be married. It felt like, "If my own family won't talk to me about it, how likely is it that I'll be in a relationship with someone within my community?" When my family did start to talk about it, it was assumed I'd only be with someone who was disabled. By my late twenties I was asked, "Haven't you ever met any disabled men you'd like to be with?"'

As Dhanda found, when the world tells you that being disabled means you'll never be in a loving relationship, it's easy to start believing it ourselves. Whether it's only seeing non-disabled women on dating shows or family asking about our sibling's new partner but not ours, other people's assumptions about disability and relationships naturally impact how optimistic we feel about our own love lives. This doesn't even need to be an explicit 'I'll die alone with my cat eating my corpse' fear but just a nagging pull of self-doubt. That you are less attractive or desirable than women without disabilities. That you are somehow 'too much'. That a partner would be a saint for 'taking you on'. Add it all up and it's no wonder many of us internalize the idea that health conditions or disability are not worthy parts of who we are that a future partner will love but an embarrassing burden it's best to hide. These insecurities can feel all the louder in the early days of dating. At a time when you're trying to show someone you are Actually Gorgeous and Fun, it can feel vulnerable – or even shameful – to show them you are a real human being with needs. In the brutal world of the dating market, it can seem as if being disabled automatically sends us down the ranking.

It's not as if these are always irrational thoughts. The reality is that, for all the wonderful prospective partners out there, there are some people – OK, predominantly men – who still hold deeply ableist attitudes towards disabled women. We have all known the lads who laugh with their friends at the bar as they point to the 'pig in the wheelchair' or the 'nice guys' who overlook women with disabilities as if they were invisible ('I see you like my sister'). It means disabled women can often go into dating being self-conscious that many non-disabled people have preconceived or stereo-typical ideas about disability. To the wrong ears, telling someone 'I'm disabled' can feel like telling them 'I'm sexless and tragic'.

When I was in my late twenties, I remember being moved by a guy who asked me out while saying his mum died from a disability – which you wouldn't think was the sexiest come-on but it worked at the time. Maybe I have low stand-ards. That's for my therapist to decide. Really, I think I felt a sense of relief or at least an understanding, as if I were speaking a foreign language and he had told me he was able to translate. If I'm honest, this low-key unease with potential dates has followed me over the years. Throughout any conversation, every flirtation, their potential reaction to my disability has lurked at the back of my mind, like a dormant Second World War grenade buried in the backyard. It is hard to have faith that someone out there will want you just as you are when you've grown up in a culture which says that they won't.

For broadcaster Nikki Fox, these worries impacted her approach to dating for over a decade. When she was younger, Fox, who has muscular dystrophy and dyslexia, enjoyed going on regular dates. But when she became more visibly disabled in her twenties, her confidence around relationships plummeted. 'I liked how I looked standing. A washboard stomach. A good, enormous arse. When I was still walking, I dated a lot. A lot. Then between the age of twenty-five and forty, when I'd started using a scooter, I didn't have a relationship at all. It was partly because I felt I had to concentrate on my career – I was worried about my disability affecting it – but it was also, I guess, that I lost confidence in my sexiness. I used to get a lot of attention from boys when I was walking around. When I got in a scooter, it was dry as a fucking desert.

'There was this guy I was seeing in my thirties – not really seeing but, y'know, seeing. I remember I didn't really want him to see me in the scooter. I couldn't wrap my head around it. I was coming to terms myself with being able to do less for myself. Would a partner not find that sexy? It was like I worried the less I could do for myself, the less sexy I would be to other people.

'I used to go to this local pub for karaoke and there was a manager there, quite creepy, who would flirt with me [when I was still walking]. I saw him again on my thirtieth birthday on a night out and he asked why I was using a scooter now. Then he looked me dead in the eye and said: "I really don't fancy you in that. It's like something a granny would use." It felt like being hit by a ton of bricks. I don't know why the opinion of an unattractive, sweaty man got to me but it did. It was like he was verbalizing my fears. And then I got so drunk. By 10.30 p.m., I was projectile-vomiting over my best friend's husband's suede shoes with two balloons coming out my scooter. It was at that point that I said, "Fuck it." I realized I had a lot of love to give and that I just needed to find the right person. Which I now have. Now, I know that my husband doesn't care about doing things for me. If anything, it brings us closer.'

Actor Cherylee Houston MBE, who uses a wheelchair due to Ehlers–Danlos syndrome and produced a BBC Radio 4 series about disability and dating, is familiar with these feelings herself. 'I think dating is the area where we question ourselves the most. We can become entirely comfortable with our disability in our friendships and social relationships, but can be unsure of ourselves with dating. I've felt really underconfident about my value, like I don't have the same worth as my non-disabled peers. I think this stems from how we're perceived in the media as much as by dates themselves, to be honest – the prejudice that's reflected back at us. That's not my fault. That's society's fault.

'I remember arranging to meet a guy who I had been talking to online. I suggested meeting in town underneath a big wheel and used the opportunity to mention my disability by sending an email saying "speaking of wheels . . ." I got an email back saying, "I'm really sorry but my sister's handi-capped herself and that's not something I'd want to do in life."'

As Houston found, the dominance of online dating over the last decade has added another layer of complexity to dating with a disability. While 'I hate the apps' is a sen-timent many non-disabled women can identify with, for those of us with health conditions, online dating can throw up a sea of dilemmas (read: existential crises). If I show my disability in the photo, will I get any matches? If I crop my wheelchair or hearing aid out of the image, will I be accused of lying? How long into messaging someone do I mention my disability? And how do I do it? Online dating can be great for some disabled women and non-binary people – not least because it can be a more accessible way of meeting people – but research suggests apps are far from equal. Only just over 5 per cent of people in the UK have been on a date with a disabled person they met through an online dating site or app like Tinder, according to a survey by Scope.[16] Younger generations are not necessarily making as much progress as we'd hope. A survey by Tinder in 2023 into the dating attitudes of 18–25-year-olds found that, while Gen Z are generally progressive in their relationship choices, only half of users would consider dating someone disabled or neurodivergent.[17] I doubt disabled women need a study to confirm that. Most of us with a disability can recount stories of awkward situations or outright prejudice online, from men opening the chat with questions about how our disability affects sex to being ghosted once you mention your condition.

Comedian Rosie Jones, who has cerebral palsy, knows this well. 'Disabled people and sex . . . it feels like it's still quite a taboo subject, doesn't it? I was recently asked what makes dating harder, my disability, or my sexuality (I identify as a lesbian) . . . and I said, "Neither, the thing that makes dating hardest is my personality." My disability has meant that, when it comes to dating, I am insanely picky. I recently blocked someone on a dating app because she said her hobby was "crocheting" . . . which is not one of my proudest moments. I will never simply "settle". I often do not have control of my body, but the thing I can control is who has my body.

'I no longer use online dating . . . but when I did use it I was very conflicted. I never knew whether I should disclose my disability when I was talking to somebody. I never wanted to blurt it out as the first thing, "HELLO I AM DISABLED", but then, if I didn't tell them at the beginning, I got worried that they would accuse me of catfishing them because I was withholding a big thing. I also found that if I put that I was disabled in my bio I would receive little to no matches. It's easy to dismiss somebody you don't know and I think by disclosing that I have a disability from the get-go, it's enough for people to not want to give me the time of day.'

Despite the difficulties she's encountered on the apps, Jones has gradually noticed progress in attitudes offline. 'When I started going to clubs, about fifteen years ago, I'd be hit on by men who would fetishize me. "Will you dribble on my cock?" is a question I've been asked too many times. I always thought that sex for me would have to be a kinky, sordid affair, and love would never be an option. But more recently, this never happens, and I never feel like I'm being fetishized. Maybe it's because I'm older, wiser, and I am hanging out in more sophisticated circles, but I hope it's because we live in a wiser world. A world in which I, a thirty-something disabled lesbian, will one day marry the non-crocheting woman of her dreams!'

I reckon Jones's optimism is worth holding on to. This is not to say that disability or ableism can't be hurdles in our love lives or that a romantic relationship is always possible. You might not be in the mental space for a relationship right now. Perhaps you're not physically well enough to date. Or your health condition means you're not able to become a mum. It's natural to grieve that, not least in a society in which the relentless pursuit of a romantic partner is seen as 'normal' and any alternative way of living is assigned less value. Women in particular are still conditioned from a young age to feel that being wanted by a man is the pinnacle of life, and getting one to 'put a ring on it' is the key to fulfilment. Anyone who doesn't fit that heteronormative box can quickly feel like there's something wrong with them. This is even more the case for women with disabilities who are already fighting to 'prove' they are sexual and romantic to a culture that too often says we aren't. In this context, it's easy to get into a relentless cycle of trying to fling yourself into a relationship, or to feel shame that you aren't in one. Be kind to those thoughts, whatever form they take. It's OK not to be fussed about dating. It's OK to feel that your health has taken something from you (even temporarily) that you really wanted, and to be sad about that. It's OK to be angry at a world that still feeds non-disabled people the message that they can't see a disabled woman *that* way. It's also more than OK to focus on other ways you can nurture this part of you. Channel Miley Cyrus and send yourself flowers. Start an online relationship with a Texan trucker named Bubba. Hug your girlfriends because life partners come in many different shapes.*

And then if you are able – and crucially, want – to date, I hope you won't rule yourself out. When you've been made

* See the end of this chapter.

to feel sexless and high-maintenance, it's natural to lose some of your confidence. If you've had a few bad experiences, this is only going to be compounded. Think of it as confirmation bias: if you go into dating with low self-esteem about your value, a few bad dates can confirm your fear that that's all there will ever be. I only have to look to my disabled friends in happy relationships to know that isn't the end of the story. There are many, many people out there who couldn't care less about the way you walk, as long as you're kind and laugh at their jokes. Let finding them be fun and exciting, not a determinant of your self-worth. Intimacy, love and affection are not incompatible with disability; they sit alongside it daily, in hard kisses and first dances. I can't promise that you will meet the love of your life – that's entirely down to chance, for non-disabled people too. But I can say with 100 per cent certainty that your disability will not matter to the right person – and they will be lucky to love you.

Now in her forties, Houston has put worries about dating behind her. 'As time has gone on, and I've been in loving relationships, I realize that actually my disability has nothing to do with my role within that relationship. I've been with my boyfriend, Toby, now for nine years and the only way disability impacts on that is caused by inaccessible buildings we want to go on a date to, or other people's attitudes . . . I don't think the fact I use a wheelchair has any semblance in our daily lives until we leave the house and meet the world.

'I remember early on in my relationship with Toby, I was in so much pain and had been for days. It was so bad that I couldn't move. After listening to my pain update he said to me, "I've just stubbed my toe." It was a great way to show me that my disability wasn't an issue for him.'

'Can u hav sex?'

When I was in sixth-form, a policeman came to my school to talk about consent. This being the early 2000s, consent workshops were focused less on how to have healthy personal relationships and more the rapist in the bushes. A hundred teenage girls sat cross-legged in a large gym hall, we listened as the policeman went through the basics of self-defence. If a man was trying to touch us in a way we didn't want, the lesson went, we had a last resort: kick him in the balls. Noticing the disabled girl in the corner, the policeman looked at me and paused. Reaching in his trouser pocket, he handed me a whistle: 'Just blow on this hard.' Good life advice.

For most of us growing up, sex education at school was less than comprehensive. Probably a banana and a condom. But if you have a disability, it's likely conversations about sex and consent were even more scarce. Evidence shows that young people with disabilities often miss out on sex education altogether compared to their non-disabled peers; a 2010 report by Leonard Cheshire found almost 50 per cent of disabled people surveyed said that they received no relationship and sex education (RSE) at school,[18] with no research bothering to update that figure since. Even if young women do receive standard sex ed, it's highly unlikely they'll get support tailored for their specific needs, whether that's consent information in easy-read format for girls with learning disabilities or advice on contraception that works for particular health conditions.

Kit Bithell, formerly an education and wellbeing specialist with Brook, a nationwide sexual health charity, who has ME and is neurodivergent, says there are multiple reasons disabled girls miss out on sex education. 'Disabled young people are more likely to be pulled out of RSE compared to non-disabled young people, as learning about sex and relationships may be seen as "inappropriate" or something that they "aren't going to need". Because disabled women are infantilized, talking about sex can often be dismissed by parents, carers, teachers and healthcare professionals in an attempt to "guard" them from knowledge of safer sex and relationships.

'If a young person was educated in a special school prior to the introduction of the RSHE curriculum in 2020, it is more likely that they may have never received sex education. That can mean they leave school with huge gaps in their knowledge, not just about sex, but also basic subjects such as puberty. That can then be compounded by discrimination they receive from other services. Our education specialists see young disabled women [who] are given hormonal contraception to prevent them from becoming pregnant without being told what it is or giving their consent.

'If disabled teenage girls are regularly absent from school, they may also miss out on sex education that way. As RSE doesn't contribute to final grades, it can often be seen as something it is "OK to miss", so catch-up options may not be provided and pupils may even be pulled out of RSE in order to focus on "core" subjects. Communication can also be an issue. If a disabled teenage girl has a health condition which may be exacerbated by sexual activity, they may be uncomfortable and feel too exposed asking questions in class about how someone with these conditions can have sex. Teachers may also not have the skills, knowledge and training to provide the answers disabled teenage girls need. This can all have a massive impact on how disabled women approach sex and relationships.'

Zoe Lloyd, campaign manager at the charity Enhance UK which runs the Undressing Disability campaign, and who herself has rheumatoid arthritis, points out this all has a real knock-on effect on disabled women's future sex lives. 'There are some sex educators who are tailoring their programmes to disabled people, like Split Banana,[19] who run workshops with young people and train educators, but there's still a serious lack of disability representation in a lot of sex ed materials. If you're a disabled teenager in a lesson and you don't see anyone in the videos that looks like you, you may think that sex isn't meant for you. You may switch off and miss out on important information. Or it may prevent you asking questions of the teacher that are more specific to your needs.

'We know that this exclusion goes on beyond the classroom. When it comes to disabled women who rely on care staff, there's a lack of training for carers in how best to support their clients to fulfil their sexual needs. Many care providers don't consider disabled people's need for relationships and sexual expression, so these topics are never addressed here either. That's why we started sexual expression training for care homes, the first ever accredited course of its nature.

'There are real consequences to this exclusion. Disabled women are three times more likely to be sexually abused. People who missed out on sex ed may not realize what a healthy relationship is, or have their vulnerability taken advantage of. Or some disabled women feel they have to put up with someone's bad behaviour, especially if that person cares for them. Lack of sex education can also result in unwanted pregnancy and STIs. Some research shows teenage girls with learning disabilities are more likely to fall pregnant compared to non-disabled teenagers.'

For broadcaster Samantha Renke, who has a brittle bone condition, sex ed at school reinforced ableist attitudes – something that's carried on into her adult life. 'I have a vivid memory of sitting in one of the English classrooms waiting for sex education. You could feel the awkward atmosphere from all the kids. We must've been thirteen or fourteen. I remember feeling like I wanted the ground to swallow me up because the kids had already started asking me intrusive questions about my own capabilities for sex as a disabled person and a wheelchair user, and as someone who is petite stature with brittle bones. One girl asked me: "Can you kiss a boy or would you break your jaw?" Another mocking insult was: "If you had sex, the penis would come up through your mouth." The sex education, if you could call it that, was generic and done with haste. And only added to my own unanswered questions.

'Growing up, I placed my self-worth on my ability or not to have a sexual relationship. I would spend hours feeling sad, anxious, confused, scared and lonely, thinking a lot about it. I felt like it was just another human experience I was never going to have because of my disability. Still to this day, I have low self-esteem when it comes to relationships. Strangers, mostly men, ask if I can have sex or if my genitalia work. I've had my wheelchair turned into a weapon so someone could grope me. I've been fetishized. I've been a one-night stand, a friend, but never a long-term girlfriend. I've actually had therapy about it.

'I wish we had the courage to educate society on disability, sex, relationships, motherhood and more. I think if we taught from a young age about different bodies and the importance of being intimate, not just penetrative sex, my life and many others would be a lot easier.'

I can't help but think Renke is right. All of us – disabled and non-disabled – would be better off if we expanded our definition of who exactly can experience sexual pleasure and what that pleasure might look like. After all, the prejudice that is levied at disabled women's sex lives is in many ways a specific version of wider attempts to control and judge female sexuality. In a society that elevates white, thin, non-disabled bodies, many of us can feel that we have to adhere to certain feminine standards to 'deserve' a healthy intimate relationship or be classed as a sexual being at all.

At the same time, women are still taught to prioritize men's sexual satisfaction and to put our own on the back burner. Look at the age-old issue of women faking orgasms. A study in 2017 of two thousand men and women across Europe and the US found 68 per cent of women admitted to faking an orgasm with their partner at some point, compared to just 27 per cent of men.[20] For women and non-binary people with disabilities and health conditions, sidelining our own sexual desires can take many additional forms. If your depression means you don't currently have a sex drive, you might feel obliged to have sex with your partner anyway. If chronic pain makes certain sexual positions uncomfortable, you could feel unable to tell your partner you'd prefer something else. Any feelings of self-doubt will only encourage this; if we worry our disability means we're not as desirable as other women or are 'harder work', we're more likely to quietly put up with things we otherwise wouldn't.

Journalist Lara Parker spent years feeling ashamed about how endometriosis affects her sexually – until she found the right partner. 'Dating as a straight woman who can't have penetrative sex and who is often in a lot of pain is definitely something that brought a lot of heartbreak with it. For a long time, I internalized every shit-bag named Jake who "just couldn't handle me" as being my fault, as if it meant that I were unlovable or undesirable in any way. There were so, so many nights when I honestly cried myself to sleep because I was so convinced that no one would ever be able to love me for me and the way that I worked. Then my ex-boyfriend came along. We started as friends and then dated for nearly four years. The relationship was tumultuous and at times painful but it taught me something very important which is that when you really love someone, nothing else really matters. Now, that doesn't mean it's going to be easy. But honestly, when it came to dating, I realized that if the only way a guy could figure out how to fuck me is by sticking his dick inside me, why would I want to waste my time with him anyway?'

As Parker discovered, penetration is far from the only way to have sex. Emilie Cousins, programme manager for Fumble, a youth charity that specializes in relationships and sex education, and who themself has long Covid, stresses there are many different ways to be intimate that work for our disabilities – with a partner or by ourselves. 'There are lots of scripts in society about what sex should be, for example, penis-in-vagina penetration, and both people simultaneously finishing with an orgasm. Not everyone is going to enjoy this particular type of sex – not just people with disabilities but also [many] women and people with a vagina who can't orgasm from penetration, or LGBTQ+ people. Try to step back from the idea of "normal sex" and think about what sexual intimacy you enjoy and want with someone else. Instead of asking yourself the question "How do I overcome my disability so that I can have sex?", start thinking about what types of sexual intimacy feel good and give you pleasure, with the body you have. The question "How do I enjoy sexual intimacy?" is a much better place to begin.

'There are so many different ways to enjoy sexual intimacy: for example, massaging, mutual masturbation, having a bath together. If you're unsure what you want from sexual intimacy and what you enjoy, masturbation is a great place to start, whether you're in a relationship or not. Sex toys aren't essential for self-pleasure, but if you're curious, there's a lot to choose from. There are sex toys specifically made for people with disabilities, such as vibrators with buttons that are bigger, embossed and easy to find, making it easier for people with visual impairment, or toys that are specifically designed for people with limited hand movement or chronic fatigue. Beyond sexual intimacy, there are lots of non-physical ways to be intimate with your partner. Romantic and emotional intimacy can be just as pleasurable and important: for example, having shared interests and hobbies, feeling supported by each other, or watching favourite TV shows together.

'We talk a lot about not pressuring another person into doing something sexual that they're not sure about or don't want, but there can also be an element of self-pressure. This especially surfaces when we're (maybe subconsciously) trying to match up to "normal sex". It can take a lot of time, intention and work to unlearn all the norms surrounding sex, but it's worth it when you reach a place where you're enjoying and relaxing into fun sexual intimacy. Sex should be fun.'

In a way, the pressure Cousins speaks of is reminiscent of what we've discussed in previous chapters. Whether it's the pull to exhaust ourselves working nine to five, leaving our cane at home so no one sees it, or wincing through a sexual position that's unsafe for us, there is often a nagging pressure to do whatever everyone else is doing.* For our disabled bodies to conform to non-disabled people's. To be . . . 'normal'. Too often, we are conditioned to see being different – or simply doing things differently – as a negative when rationally it is anything but. That's the case with intimacy too. Great sex – and a great relationship – is inventive, communicative and can take whatever shape

* Or what we *think* they are doing.

works for you.* Whether it's sex with a partner, masturbation, or an online fetish involving antique buttons, there are many wonderful ways to make sex accessible.

Cousins says a good place to start is doing some research and thinking about what would help you practically. 'Get creative! It could involve sex toys, lube, cushions, chairs, and many other things. It could be that certain positions feel easier or more comfortable, or that you need breaks. It could be that sometimes you have a flare-up and, for example, your hand movement is especially restricted, so you can't enjoy fingering for a time. That's OK! This is a chance to change things up and think about other types of sexual intimacy that you could try instead: for example, using a sex toy that allows for low movement and is easier on your hand. Don't push through pain. Pain is your body's way of telling you that something's wrong. There will be sexual intimacy that works for you, is pain-free and, even better, is pleasurable! It just may take some time to figure it out.

'Communicate with your sexual partner. Tell them about what you've figured out, what you'd like to try, and what feels good sexually. Talking about sex can feel really hard, and this can get even harder if you have the added layer of disability. So be gentle with yourself if you're struggling, and try not to pile on the pressure. If it feels easier to have

* And, of course, that includes not wanting sex at all.

the first few conversations over [phone] messages, then do that. Remember, you have the right to safe sexual pleasure, regardless of your disability, whether that's self-pleasure or partnered sex. If the other person isn't receptive to what you need to stay safe while having sex, then that's not OK and it isn't safe to have sex with them.'

Actor Jameela Jamil, who has Ehlers–Danlos syndrome, says she goes into every relationship knowing how well a partner should treat her. 'I'm just not an athletic shag. I don't think it's technically a symptom of EDS, but I'd venture to call it one. Keep all sex swings and BDSM away from me please. I didn't [feel pressure growing up around sex]. I had known since I was nine I had EDS, and I was maybe twenty-two when I started having sex, so I was very self-preservation [focused] already. I had multiple full-time jobs and just didn't have time to get sicker than necessary!

'[When it comes to dating], a chronic condition like this requires planning, and excessive safety measures. I can't just "go with the flow". I can't do a lot of active things or go out clubbing all night in heels. I have always been lucky to only date men who love bed as much as I do and who never make me feel bad for not being able to always join in. I really truly believe that if you're not the sort of person who would walk out on someone if they had a health reason for not being able to do something, then you shouldn't tolerate intolerance in your partner. I would never make a person

with a bad back have sex with me in the shower or something and so I expect reciprocity of care and respect.'

Care and respect? They are good things to expect from
a sexual partner, I think. I'm a firm believer that the bar
we set for our Uber driver should not be higher than the
one we set for the person inside of us. Still, finding the
confidence to seek all we've discussed – communication,
satisfaction, consideration – from a partner is not always
easy. Nor is it necessarily simple to feel connected to your
sexuality in a culture that likes to desexualize you. After
all, the way in which sex education excludes and stereotypes disabled women is not confined to the classroom; it is
replicated in many forms throughout our adult lives, from
popular culture, sexual health services, to ableist dates. But
I hope the last few pages have shown this is far from the
end of the story. Disabled women are carving out our own
ways to find pleasure and intimacy, simultaneously redefining one-dimensional sex and reclaiming our sexualities with the support of each other.

This isn't only about having a healthy relationship with
someone else, I think, but a healthy relationship with ourselves. When you're disabled, you often have to endure
other people's intrusive touch. Doctors prod your skin.
Care workers might help you dress. At the same time, a
variety of symptoms can rear their head from day to
day, our joints or muscles behaving in any way they wish
without granting us a choice. It can feel sometimes as if

your flesh is an enemy working against you, that your nerve endings are somehow made solely for pain. In this context, physical intimacy isn't only a form of welcome pleasure – it can feel like a way to take back control of your own body. This body, that they so desperately want to convince us is made wrong, that is humming with sparks and fucking fire.

Friends with benefits

When it comes to relationships, society likes to rank friendship below romantic partners. Shops sell anniversary cards to celebrate marriages, not mates. We throw an expensive reception to mark committing to a lover, not a best friend for life. This is despite the fact it is these platonic relationships – unconditional, decades-long – that can be some of the most meaningful of our lives. If you're disabled, it isn't just that society doesn't value our friendships – it often doesn't think we have them at all. The same cultural norms we have seen paint disability as inherently tragic and abnormal perpetuate the myth that disabled women don't have happy relationships or socialize like other people. I imagine many of us who are visibly disabled have at some point been on a night out with friends minding our own business only for a stranger to touch our arm and congratulate us. 'Good for you, getting out!' they cry, as if I'm a prisoner of war escaping a barbed-wire compound rather than a millennial who stumbled thirty yards to the nearest All Bar One. I sometimes think that half the reason I can turn up to a friend's birthday drinks and be blocked by a single step to the bar is because it just never occurred to the manager a disabled person would ever be there to need a ramp. A viral tweet in 2018 summed this attitude up perfectly: 'Disabled parking should only be valid during business hours 9 to 5 Monday to Friday. I cannot see any reason why people with genuine disabilities would be out beyond these times.' As Jennifer Lee Rossman replied to the applause of 400,000 'likes', 'We're disabled. We're not werewolves.'[21]

These ideas are pernicious, not only infiltrating social attitudes but even affecting government policy. The underfunding of the social care system over the last decade has seen disabled care users have their day-to-day lives curtailed. Many are allocated care solely for personal needs, like getting dressed, and have had 'social hours' like support to see friends removed. Others have been given early 'bedtime' slots because no carer is available to help them later. Some are forced to bed at 5 p.m.[22] Meanwhile, cuts to the benefit system mean tens of thousands of disabled people have had their adapted cars taken away in recent years,[23] leaving many housebound with no way to go out with loved ones. The factors behind these policies are complex but attitudes to disability are surely part of the picture. It is hard to imagine policy-makers expecting non-disabled people to go to bed before the sun sets or to just stop leaving their house. They wouldn't – because they have been raised with the belief that, unlike disabled people, 'normal people' have social lives and relationships.

In the face of this, placing value on disabled people's friendships can feel particularly important. I'm not going to suggest that going to the pub is a political act (will my wine come with a tax break?) but countering the idea that we don't want to is. Let's call it the politics of disabled joy, where every time we laugh and dance it is an act of defiance against the idea that disability means we should be miserable. One thing I hope this book shows is that whether it is our careers, body image or relationships, there is enormous humour, community and love in the disabled experience. When I think about happy moments with friends over the years, my disability is essentially a supporting character: it is never the main plot line but is often lurking in the background. The friend who borrowed a builder's ramp from roadworks in central London to help me get up a kerb to the restaurant. The pub crawl that descended into a 1980s sports bar because venues without sticky floors don't necessarily have wheelchair access. The care packages that arrived through the post in the first months of my illness: a magazine, a chocolate bar, and an unspoken 'I'm thinking of you'.

Broadcaster Sophie Morgan, who became paralysed in her late teens, counts her friends as some of the most important relationships in her life and often leans on them for support with her health. 'My disability means that my friends often have to help me and that's OK, it brings us closer. They carry spare catheters in their handbags for me in case I need them. They even carry me if we get to inaccessible spaces.

Once, me and two friends were laughing so much I fell off my chair. When we eventually stopped laughing long enough for them to help lift me off the ground, one friend picked up one leg, the other friend picked up the other and, without checking, one walked one way and one walked in the opposite direction, making me do the splits. It was so funny we all fell over laughing again.'

Morgan's splits remind me of a running joke I've had with a friend who would always end up being the one to help me put my coat on after a meal out. He would consistently fail to get the sleeves right and came to dread the sight of it, but would plough on, with game commitment. (I can't help it that I make innovative fashion choices.) There is an intimacy to these moments; an entirely mundane act that is also about trust, honesty and acceptance. There is no pressure to hide away your disability from these friends or to make it the central part of your relationship either. It's just there, like sugar on a doughnut.

It's not always simple, though. The disabled joy I spoke of at the start of this section is very real but that isn't to say it's easy to feel. When you're going through health problems or dealing with the day-to-day hassle of being disabled in an inaccessible world, there are barriers that mean it can be difficult to connect with friends. For a start, many of the public venues designed for socializing in the UK aren't accessible for disabled people. A survey of pubs and bars by Euan's Guide in 2023 found only 25 per cent of disabled respondents said these spaces had 'good' accessibility,[24] while Leonard Cheshire reports eight in ten[25] disabled people face difficulties going to bars and pubs. Those after-work drinks with colleagues are a no-go if the venue is the top floor of a pub without a lift. Things can be even harder for gay disabled people: approximately 40 per cent of the LGBTQ+ community identify as having a disability but a survey by ParaPride found there's not a single LGBTQ+ space in the UK that's fully accessible.[26] The knock-on effect is a kind of all-year-round lockdown only for disabled people.* Research by the Belonging Forum in 2024 found a quarter of people with disabilities 'never go' to a pub, bar or coffee shop with their friends, compared to 17 per cent of the general population.[27]†

It isn't just steps that keep us out. Social attitudes can be just as excluding as physical barriers: research by Scope[28] shows one in five disabled people (23 per cent) avoid going out to social gatherings following negative attitudes and behaviour about their disability. Younger disabled people are more than twice as likely to avoid socializing

---

* Of course, many disabled people have had an extended 'lockdown' since 2020 due to the ongoing pandemic. The removal of corona-virus protection measures – from free testing, mask mandates, to poor ventilation – in recent years means some clinically vulnerable people are still shut out of busy public spaces, like pubs, restaurants and festivals, long after the general population were able to 'return to normal'.

† This increases to 32 per cent for those aged forty-five to fifty-four who have a disability.

outside their homes (35 per cent) as disabled people who are fifty-five or over (15 per cent). That's a remarkable admission when you stop to think about it: more than a third of young disabled people feel they have to actively avoid going out because they're afraid of what the public will say or do. And yet negative attitudes aren't just an issue from people we don't know – but also from those we do. Maybe you're Deaf and it's hard to lip-read in large groups at work because colleagues don't look at you when they speak. Or you have chronic fatigue and friends struggle to understand why 'you're just tired all the time'. Many of these attitudes are of course not intentionally hurtful – more a kind of ignorance or thoughtlessness – but that doesn't mean it's not hard to be on the receiving end. I think this can get more complicated still if our friendship circle is full of non-disabled people – especially when we're young. At this point in our lives, most of our mates' bodies will still be in A+ condition and their only experience with being unwell (hopefully) is a bout of the flu. When we're struggling with symptoms that those around us have never felt, it can naturally impact our relationships with them, especially if our health has changed since we met. Friends might not know what to say. Or may utter something clumsy or upsetting. Some will be there when we need support. Others might fall away.

Despite how close she is with her friends, when Sophie Morgan first became disabled, she found it hard to connect with her non-disabled mates. 'When I was first injured at eighteen years old, none of my friends were disabled and I felt very isolated. It was hard keeping up both physically and emotionally, and although I didn't admit it, I struggled to relate to them and their non-disabled lives at times. Being a wheelchair user and a paraplegic, my life, with all its ups and downs, had overnight become so different to my friends'. Thanks to a charity for people with spinal injury, I made friends with other young people who had also been through similar trauma and found a powerful connection with them, but it would be a few more years before I actually made true lasting friendships with people who happened to have disabilities but also the sorts of shared interests I looked for in all my friendships. Friends are so important to me, and while today some of my best friends don't have disabilities, I know how to ask for help and lean on them when I need them.'

As Morgan has found, trying to be honest with our loved ones about how we're feeling – and what we might need from them – is one of the most useful things we can do. I think many of us, regardless of health, can struggle to articulate our feelings to friends during a hard time, or feel obliged to downplay our (more batshit) emotions. When a friend asks, 'How are you?' many of us plump for a low-maintenance 'Fine' even if we're very much not. This pull for fine-ness can be even stronger if you're living with chronic conditions and trying to navigate friendships with non-disabled mates. We can feel self-conscious about being 'too much' as if we're 'going on' about our illness, or struggle to explain symptoms that seem alien to someone who's never had them. If we do share honestly with a friend without diluting the toughest parts, we can end up having to make the other, healthy person feel better about the situation. Sometimes, it feels simpler to just keep things to ourselves. In an age when much of our connection is on social media, hiding the impact of our health has become even easier behind a screen. 'How are you?' 'Really good, actually!' I type, as blood gushes from my decapitated skull.

Journalist Hannah Jane Parkinson, who has bipolar and ADHD, counts herself as lucky to have a wide circle of friends who 'I can be mostly honest with and who support me immensely'. But she admits her mental health can be 'intensely isolating'. 'The nature of depressive episodes, in particular, usually means that one has awful self-esteem, so often I withdraw because I think I'm a burden or that I won't be good enough company for people. The other thing with depression is that it often means sleeping a lot, or existing in a sort of catatonic fog, which means I don't leave the house. And obviously if I'm sleeping all day I end up missing plans and engagements. Then it becomes a cycle where the more I withdraw the worse I feel. And while I can talk to people about how I'm feeling, I think the severity of it can be quite hard to convey. As for the ADHD, that's something that means day-to-day I'm quite bad at responding to messages. I'm late a lot of the time, which is immensely rude, and I feel permanently guilty about it, but I basically have no sense of time and I really struggle with a lot of basic domestic tasks too, which means I very rarely invite people round. And I have a huge amount of shame around this.

'If I'm depressed I can also drink too much and send, like, 2,000-word texts, which is . . . a bad idea. It's definitely not always easy to be around people in various states of mental distress, which is why I feel such loyalty to the people who are supportive. I really appreciate when I'm pulling out of a down phase and I will do simple things one-on-one with friends as I'm getting back on my feet. Walks in the park, or when I was in hospital and was allowed out in the days, my friend David and I going to the pub to watch the football. But at the moment, for instance, I'm not doing well and I do feel . . . "Oh God, why do they stick around?" I must really be amazing the rest of the time.'

If you have a friend with a health condition, you are not The Worst Person Alive if you don't know how to handle it. There's no set right thing to do, no magic words to say; you know your friend best and what works for one person won't necessarily for another. But you can never go wrong by simply thinking about them and what they might need. Check meeting places you suggest are accessible for their disability. Offer to go round to their place if it's easier. Keep inviting them even if they often say no; an 'I know you might not be well enough to come but just wanted to let you know we all miss you' goes a very long way. Understand health conditions can be fluctuating and that they may have to pull out last minute, even on your birthday. That they've had to cancel meeting up is no reflection on you – but how you react about it is. Ask how they're doing and keep asking. A chronic condition rarely goes away but friends' interest does. Do all the little things you always have done; WhatsApp that TV recommendation, tag them in that meme that you know would make them laugh. They are still the person they always were (maybe just a bit more sore and tired).

It can be lonely to be disabled or ill. That is not a revolutionary thing to say and yet it is something that we often struggle to admit out loud. There's still a stigma attached to the idea of loneliness, particularly amongst young people, as if admitting we are lonely sometimes means saying we're Friendless Losers rather than just human beings with completely natural needs. In recent years, loneliness has become an epidemic across the general population. In the UK alone, 25 million people report they are occasionally, sometimes or often lonely, according to the Campaign to End Loneliness.[29] But if you're disabled, you're even more likely to be affected. Research from Sense[30] in 2021 shows the scale of this: almost two-thirds of disabled people (61 per cent) are chronically lonely, meaning they feel lonely 'always' or 'often'. The picture is even worse when it comes to younger disabled people; seven in ten (70 per cent) of those surveyed between the ages of sixteen and twenty-four said they were lonely.

So, what's causing this crisis? For some disabled people, loneliness stems from social isolation – that is, not regularly coming into contact with other people. Those of us who have a disability are less likely to have significant friendships: 14 per cent of disabled people have no close friends at all, compared to 9 per cent without a disability, according to research by the Belonging Foundation in 2024.[31] Disabled people aren't just less likely to have good mates to spend time with – we're less likely to even see acquaintances or strangers. A study by Scope in 2017 found that, in a typical day, one in eight disabled people spend less than half an hour interacting with another person.[32] That seems shocking – and it is – but in some ways, it's not at all surprising when you consider how segregated many disabled people still are from the rest of society. I don't just mean the way most restaurants don't have hearing loops or that the local bus only has a single wheelchair space. I mean the way much of the non-disabled public actively keep their distance from disabled people. Research shows eight out of ten people in Britain have never invited a disabled person to a social occasion and half have never started a conversation with someone disabled.[33] We might hope that younger generations have more progressive outlooks in their social lives but it can actually be the opposite. Millennials are twice as likely as boomers to feel awkward around people with disabilities, while a fifth of 18–34-year-olds admit to avoiding interactions entirely because they're unsure how to communicate.[34] The impact of all this is brutal. The Sense study[35] found two-thirds (70 per cent) of disabled people say that social isolation is affecting their mental health and wellbeing, with two in five (40 per cent) reporting an impact on their physical health.

Dr Sula Windgassen, a health psychologist who previously had bladder pain syndrome herself, says there are multiple reasons disabled people are more likely to experience loneliness. 'In our society, it can feel hard for anyone to feel connected but that can especially be the case when a chronic condition or disability is involved. Our ability to participate in everyday social activities can be more impeded, whether because of practical barriers like limited toilets, a lack of wheelchair access or lack of money, or because of social attitudes like being guilted if we have to leave a party early or can't drink. When you're the only one or the minority experiencing this, it can be incredibly lonely.

'People who need to pace their energy or whose bodies don't allow them to "keep pushing" can feel an inherent sense of failing when out socializing. It's really isolating to want to be able to participate and not be able to because your health stops you. Many patients of mine talk about fearing going out in case they are not on top form and their friends see them as a "downer". They then might try to limit their socializing to only when they know they won't be at all affected by symptoms, or minimally so. They feel they have to put on a brave face and spare people from their vulnerability. Although intended to be protective, this can have the counterproductive impact of being even more isolating and withdrawing.'

As Windgassen says, disabled people are often physically isolated from social settings – but we don't have to be alone to feel lonely. Everyone can identify with the cliché of being in a room full of people and yet still feeling alone. Rosie Weatherley, Information Content Manager at Mind, who herself has bipolar disorder type II, says that this sense of emotional loneliness can be particularly common for disabled women. 'Having a physical or mental health condition can be perceived as a barrier to connection by those around us. We might end up feeling invisible to people we meet, or that we've been passed over due to stigma about disability and unchecked, inaccurate assumptions about who we are and what we want. It can be incredibly hurtful and insulting. Repeated rejections can harden our hearts, making it more difficult to be optimistic about, or continue to hope to develop, more intimate relationships.

'Loneliness can also manifest within close relationships we already have. Feeling dismissed, misunderstood or unseen by the people in our lives can leave us feeling lonely. If you don't feel like you are truly known and accepted for who you are, or your relationships depend on only sharing certain parts of yourself, that can be very lonely too. Your relationships might also be affected if a partner, child or relative is deeply involved in managing your condition or supports you with daily living stuff. That type of intimacy can change the dynamic of the relationship into something that leaves you feeling unfulfilled, unseen, or unable to give what you want to give to it. For example, you might find yourself feeling desexualized if your romantic partner is heavily involved in your personal care. Or that the caretaking, nurturing roles within your parent–child relationship feel reversed.'

The solutions to this are clearly at the societal level: from cultural change that would help non-disabled people grow up with a healthier view of disability in order to see disabled people as equals, friends and partners, to changes to infrastructure, such as making social venues, offices and transport more accessible, to enable disabled people to socialize like anyone else. We deserve that and it is the responsibility of non-disabled society – not us – to fix it. But in the meantime, there are many strategies we can use to support ourselves.

Windgassen has several tips for when we feel lonely. 'It sounds basic but lots of us have a tendency to fight the reality that we feel lonely and isolated. We may do this for all sorts of reasons, like the sense we're failing. If we can't acknowledge this is what we're experiencing, the feeling will show up in different ways, like restlessness or agitation. We have pretty nifty brain shortcuts to escape feelings we don't want to deal with, so we may find ourselves eating more, or compulsive busyness, or numbing out to Netflix. Instead, acknowledge to yourself how you're feeling.

'Secondly, know you're not alone or the problem. In an inherently ableist society, those with health conditions are often very practically isolated and made to feel like the "out group". As humans, we often internally attribute difficulties we encounter as being our fault or problem. Spotting this tendency and recognizing this is not a "you" problem, this is a societal issue, takes the weight off your shoulders. One thing that really helps this is being amongst others who are also impacted by similar issues, so try finding community online or in-person with other disabled people.

'Finally, experiment with opening up. It's often the norm to keep difficulties to ourselves. I often guide my patients to pick someone in their life who they feel safest with. Pick a vulnerability that it feels uncomfortable to share (it doesn't have to be the biggest vulnerability or the most uncom-fortable). Specify what you predict will happen if you share this with them. Then do it. Bite the bullet and do it. See what happens. You might want to practise saying the words out loud beforehand, especially if you want to share with someone some needs that you would like meeting in your relationship. When this inevitably doesn't end up as the cat-astrophic prediction indicated, it can give you confidence to open a little more. This takes time, care and practice. We don't need to go from completely stoic to the most open book we've ever seen. Working out what feels comfortable and, importantly, most connecting takes some experimentation. But it is worthwhile.'

When it comes to meeting more people, Weatherley recommends making the best of socializing in-person and online. 'Bringing new people into your life, or broadening your social horizons, can be a daunting prospect, even if you already know lots of people. Attending organized activities, like an art class, or volunteering can help with this; there's a structure to follow, a person in charge to focus on, and a task to distract you. Alternatively, low-key activities like coffee mornings may feel more comfortable for you.

'Online interaction can be a rewarding way to build your own sense of community, especially if your health makes it more tricky to meet up in-person. Social media platforms are certainly imperfect, so tuning in to yourself to make sure that being online is helping you is very important. It's easy to not realize you're getting overwhelmed – for example, because you find yourself providing a lot of support to others in your online community, or that you're comparing yourself to others. You could be feeling very anxious or stressed about conversations, notifications and unread messages, notice that you're increasingly disconnected from your offline life, or just burn out completely. These are signs that it's time to take a break, and rebalance your online and offline worlds. You can switch off notifications, put your device on Do Not Disturb mode, and use an app that monitors your screen time. And replace your online time with something in the physical world like reading a book or cooking a meal.'

Nowadays, it's common to hear warnings about the use of social media and the damage it can have on our wellbeing. As Weatherley points out, much of this criticism is valid: unhealthy comparisons with influencers, a filtered view of our peers, the gradual destruction of liberal democracy as we know it, etc., etc. This tension has understandably only increased as a number of big tech companies have aligned themselves with the far right and misinformation. But I think there's also some snobbery around the use of social media – snobbery that directly impacts disabled people the most. When the pandemic lockdowns ended and the world opened back up, we were told to shed our phones – that the point of human connection was hugs, not screens. Perhaps. But what if health means you can't regularly see your friends in-person? What if you have to type your anecdotes rather than say them out loud? What if you actually enjoy that? The idea that online relationships are not 'real' is a deeply ableist narrative, just as drives to 'put your phone down and meet in-person' ignore the myriad of reasons why disabled and chronically ill people may rely on the internet to form new connections or keep in touch with old ones. This is not to say that disabled people don't flourish with physical connection like anyone else or that marginalized groups aren't in fact more at risk online; research by Scope in 2023 found one in three disabled people who use social media or game online have experienced negative comments about them and their disability, shooting up to almost half of disabled 18–34-year-olds.[36] But it is to say that not everyone's circumstances are the same and there is no right way to form 'connection'. Perhaps ME means you don't have the energy to visit your uni mates across the country, so you stay in touch on a WhatsApp group. Maybe your existing friends struggle to understand your depression, so you've built a community on Instagram from mental health accounts. These relationships are no less 'real' – they can be lifelines.

For journalist and author Ione Gamble, who has Crohn's, the internet has been invaluable in helping her form friendships with other chronically ill women. 'When I was first diagnosed, I spent a lot of time looking at forums, websites and chatroom-style websites to hear about other people's experiences but most of the time people were quite different than me. [Since then], social media has come so far in terms of chronically ill communities and now it's so easy to find them. I think my generation is definitely better at seeing the import-ance in online friendships. Making chronically ill friends has really been so affirming for me. I try and personally veer away from the type of community online that focuses on health advice as often I can find that stressful but I really value con-nections in which there's already an established understand-ing of what it means to be ill. Sometimes that's as simple as having a friend who doesn't require lengthy explanations of my condition or apologies when I cancel.'

It took me until my thirties to make disabled friends. Until then, I wasn't discriminating ('eww, disabled people') – I just hadn't met any. That feels like a strange thing to say but I suppose reflects not only how isolating disability can be but how – perhaps even more so than for other minorities – there are very few spaces solely for disabled people. There are no 'disabled bars' to safely meet others in. Unless you are one of the few with a hereditary condition, your own family do not look like you or share your minority status. It's possible to exist for decades without ever coming across someone who shares a key part of your life. That only changed for me thanks to the internet; a DM with other disabled journalists that turned into friendship.

Looking back, I know having disabled friends became significantly more important to me as my health had a greater impact. I wrote earlier in this chapter that we are still the same person after we become ill or disabled and there is certainly truth in that. But it is also kind of a lie. I am not the same person I was before I fell chronically ill. None of us are. You don't set off on a trip across the Andes and come back as unbruised as when you left. The components of my personality that I have always shared with my friends are still there – politics, TV, why Benedict Cumberbatch looks like a spoon – and I love them as much as I ever did, but that is not enough now. There are other things that occupy my mind, there are new things that need saying. It is as if I am a jigsaw and there is a missing piece only someone of the same shape can fill.

Whether it's becoming a mum, losing a parent, or having a

health scare, none of our lives are static – and our friendships aren't either. If you're single but your closest friends all couple up or have kids, you'll probably end up spending more time with people who match your lifestyle. If you're a new mum, you're more likely to talk about breastfeeding with a friend who's experienced it themselves. It is one of the most human of needs to crave a shared experience. To know that someone, somewhere in the world is going through what you are. That they understand. This can be particularly vital if you're a minority like a disabled woman or non-binary person. To find 'your people' in a culture that too often isolates and others you is to be gifted a sense of belonging as much as support, like a stranger in the women's loos passing a tampon under the stall.

Gamble knows this feeling well. 'A few years ago, I wanted to do an episode for my podcast spotlighting women with chronic illness so reached out to someone on Instagram, and for the first time was sat in a room exclusively populated by women who had similar experiences to mine. We promised to keep in touch but of course in the world of chronic illness and disability that can't often be possible, so when we then ran into each other at another event later in the year it felt like fate. I remember riding home in my Uber after that evening and just feeling as though I finally had found people I could totally be at ease with. It made me feel like I finally had the freedom to truly be myself.'

As this chapter has shown, a combination of prejudice and practical barriers routinely impact disabled women's relationships. We've seen how teenage girls with disabilities often still grow up excluded from conversations about sex, the ableism that filters through dating apps as much as clubs, and the epidemic of disabled loneliness. But we have also seen the joy disabled women and non-binary people are experiencing: from loving long-term relationships, the intimacy of accessible sex and self-pleasure, to having incredible friends online and off.

In a culture where disability is still equated with misery and tragedy, and disabled women are cast as sexless and loveless, I hope the stories in this chapter can act as a middle finger to that narrative. I hope you are able to celebrate your best friendships, messy dates, and google the latest accessible vibrator. But if things are hard right now, that's more than OK too. Maybe you're spoilt for company but don't feel understood. Maybe you're by yourself, and you have been for a while. We've all been there. Please take this opportunity to wrap up in a quilt, get your favourite high-calorie snack, and think of all the disabled women out there who are in your corner. Because you are not alone. Tonight, with the pages of this book, you are surrounded by all of us (and I think I can speak for everyone here when I say we think you're pretty great).

Representation

'I often feel like I have to work harder than anyone else in the room as a disabled actress. You have to prove you can play any role regardless of disability.'
— **Ruth Madeley**

A few years ago, I was placed on a Tudor wall. As part of an exhibition for the National Trust, my portrait hung alongside Tudor paintings and 21st-century women; modern role models framed in ornate gold. I surprised myself at how moved I was by the experience. It seemed oddly poignant that someone who would have been left to beg in the street at the time that the historical portraits were painted was now hanging next to them as their equal. 'I'm the first wheelchair user to ever be on a stately-home wall,' I announced on social media. 'You are!' replied a historian. 'Other than maybe Henry VIII. When he got gout.'

I would like to say that disability representation has improved since the Tudor era, and of course it has, not least over the last two decades. Whether it is in the media, politics or the arts, there are more disabled women at the forefront of British culture than ever before. We can all celebrate this. But I know it is still far behind where it should be. From the deficit in MPs with disabilities sitting in Parliament, the marginalization of disabled models and musicians, to the stereotypical way disabled characters are often portrayed on-screen, the representation of disabled people is – despite great progress – still curtailed by a cocktail of structural barriers and prejudice.

This erasure of disability doesn't just impact the disabled women working in these industries – it can impact all of us watching at home. Disabled people are twice as likely to feel unrepresented in popular culture; a survey by the House of Commons Women and Equalities Committee in 2020[1] found one in ten people reported 'never' feeling represented in media and advertising but this rose to one in five for people with a disability. It is hard to put into words what being 'unrepresented' can do to a person, partly because the effects are rarely conscious. It is a drip, drip – a wordless message that says, 'You don't belong.' If you never or rarely see yourself reflected in television, toys or news-stands, it is hard to feel you are truly a part of society like everyone else. It is as if you are always on the outside looking in, nose pressed against the glass. This naturally has a knock-on effect not only on how minorities feel about ourselves and our place in the world but on our chance of filling those spaces in the future. We might call it the irony of inspiration: disabled people are frequently held up as 'inspirational' to the wider population, and yet we grow up in a culture that routinely shuts out the disabled public figures who could genuinely inspire us.

At the same time, poor disability representation impacts non-disabled people too – namely how they see and understand disability. Prejudice doesn't emerge from the ether. The discriminatory attitudes we've seen throughout this book – from infantilization, uselessness, to sexlessness – can be directly correlated to how disabled people are depicted by the media and the platforms we're excluded from. If you only watch stereotypical disabled characters on television, it will naturally encourage you to think disability is tragic and pitiable. If you never see a disabled cabinet minister on the news, it's easy to believe disabled people can't be authoritative or leaders.

Looking back, I realize that when I stared up at my portrait hanging on that stately-home wall, I was moved for other reasons than I first thought. It wasn't just that I was a disabled woman suddenly equal to the Tudor figures – it was that I was equal to the 21st-century ones. In that hall, disability sat proudly on display, a wheelchair user peering out alongside politicians, actors and musicians – as if I really belonged there. For some of us, that is a rare feeling. It shouldn't be.

Screen time

When I was ten, I would watch Tanni Grey-Thompson whenever a wheelchair race was on TV. I had never played sport. I found the Paralympics a bit dull, if I'm honest. But I was transfixed: it was the only time I ever saw someone on television who looked like me. Face pressed against the screen, I was like a white rhino relieved to see another horn.

By the time I was an adult, I did not need to rely on the Paralympics to see disability on my television. It was possible to switch on the news or watch a soap and to – occasionally at least – see a disabled woman staring back at me. In recent years, a surge of women with disabilities and health conditions have thrived in the entertainment industry, from critically acclaimed Liz Carr winning an Olivier Award, BAFTA-nominated Ruth Madeley getting a ramp for the Tardis in *Doctor Who*, to comedian Rosie Jones finding her place as a household name.

It has been wonderful to see – but these successes are in many ways the exception rather than the norm. In Britain, there is still a significant lack of disabled women on our screens and airwaves. Disabled people make up just 8.3 per cent of on-screen contributions in the television industry,[2] with only 6 per cent of contributors behind the scenes having a disability. Things are even worse at the top: just 3.6 per cent of executive producers are disabled.[3] This is despite the fact 16 per cent of the working population have some form of disability, and 22 per cent of viewers.

Radio is little better. Research by Ofcom in 2021[4] found only 10 per cent of the workforce in radio are disabled, while disabled people are particularly underrepresented in senior positions. Even commercial breaks exclude us. Research by Channel 4 in 2022 found just 4 per cent of adverts featured a disabled person.[5] The majority of these were older characters, while many were just supporting; staggeringly, only 1 per cent of television adverts had a disabled person playing a lead role.

And yet representation in the entertainment industry isn't just about how many disabled women are on our screens and airwaves but what they're permitted to do when they get there. On the rare occasions disabled women are featured on-screen, they are typically hired for 'disability content' and overlooked for other jobs. When I first started working in the media, I was only called by a producer when they needed to talk about disability. Fifteen years into my career, I'm still often labelled the *Guardian*'s 'disability columnist' despite this role not existing at the paper and my work focusing on politics. Call it the segregation of disabled performers: while non-disabled presenters and creatives are offered roles across a range of subjects and genres, their disabled colleagues are often pigeonholed for shows focused on disability. I realize that I always know the Paralympics have started because it is the only time I ever see more than one disabled person in a TV studio. Disabled women working in the media are essentially like

Superman and Clark Kent: you never see them in a room at the same time.

In some ways, this trend is actually getting worse. Landmark research by the Creative Diversity Network in 2021[6] – which drew on five years of data and 2.7 million contributions by the UK's main broadcasters – shows that, while there have been some small increases in the contribution of disabled people, these are limited to a few areas of production such as children's programming. In all other genres, representation is static or has been in decline. At the current rate of progress, it will take until 2041 for disabled people to be properly represented in the UK television industry.[7]

As a working actor of over two decades and co-creative lead at the Disabled Artist Networking Community, a collective of over 1,200 disabled creatives, Cherylee Houston MBE – who made British TV history in 2010 by becoming the first full-time disabled actress on *Coronation Street*[8] – has witnessed first-hand how the industry has grappled with disability representation. 'I think things have changed a lot over the past twenty years. When I first started out, there weren't really any jobs for disabled actors on television, and theatre was only really in disabled-led companies. As I started to get roles, I saw how inaccessible the industry was. I was auditioned in corridors, car parks and once in Leicester Square because I couldn't access the audition room. I once had a disabled toilet as my green room because everybody else's social spaces were at the top of a flight of stairs.

I've had jobs taken off me once they realized I had a disability, even though it was on my CV. I've been told I was a health hazard and an insurance liability.

'My experience at *Corrie*, in contrast, has been absolutely phenomenal. Before I even went in they gave me a tour around the building and we figured out which bits needed to change for my access. Years on, there's a fully wheelchair-accessible route around sets, there's flattened areas of concrete over the cobbles . . . This means that it's accessible to everyone – the camera dollies, props carrying lots of large objects, even easier for people in heels. The costume department have a heated set of clothes to go under my clothes when filming outside in winter, make-up think about how many times my hair and make-up need to be changed. When on location or filming a new set the team always consider my access, which is fantastic. After I admitted that working the full schedule was making me quite ill, they immediately moved me down to a four-day week. I even have a bed in my dressing room. I really think that *Corrie* helped pave the way for more disabled representation on television. I think we have quite a bit further to go, but it really does feel like the industry is up for the conversation, which previously always used to be a battle.'

The rate of change that Houston has seen over her career is reflective of the rapid progress the industry – and wider British society – has made over the last decade in its attitudes to disability. It was as recently as 2009 that Cerrie

Burnell – then a presenter on CBeebies, the BBC's children's channel – received a flurry of complaints from parents who objected to her being on TV. Why? Burnell has one hand. One parent wrote that her appearance 'freaked out' their child. Others lamented their child would have 'trouble sleeping' after seeing the presenter.[9]

Over fifteen years later, disabled women can largely appear on-screen without garnering official complaints from the public. You only have to click on social media whenever a famous woman with a visible disability is on television, though, to see that a significant minority in this country still has a problem with having to hear and see a confident and successful disabled woman. As Rosie Jones puts it to me: 'As a disabled comedian, I get online abuse every time I appear on television. It's simply exhausting. It seems like a large group of people desperately need to share their opinion on what I look like, what I sound like and whether or not they find me funny.'

On top of such ableist attitudes, disabled entertainers still face a myriad of practical obstacles too. Research[10] by the Sir Lenny Henry Centre for Media Diversity at Birmingham City University in 2022 into the experiences of disabled people working in television found that more than 80 per cent of those surveyed said disability had adversely affected their career. Over half (51 per cent) reported practical issues, such as not being able to drive or use certain equipment, as barriers to their employment, as well as employers failing to understand how adjustments need to be made for disabilities. Meanwhile, a study by Bournemouth University of disabled professionals in the television industry[11] found 60 per cent had experienced ableism while working or seeking work. Some reported micro-aggressions or verbal abuse, including colleagues suggesting 'what they needed to do to be cured' or their supervisor telling them disabled people shouldn't have children 'so that eventually it dies out like natural selection'.

This is all too familiar to Sophie Morgan. After getting her presenting break on Channel 4's Paralympic coverage in 2016, she has made the rare progression to being hired for broadcasting roles that aren't solely about disability issues. But as one of the only female wheelchair users in the industry, Morgan has repeatedly experienced discrimination. 'I've definitely seen progress in recent years with the generation of disabled talent coming up behind me. The industry is enabling so many of us to thrive with new initiatives and talent pathways being established. Television is such a powerful tool in the fight to change people's perceptions of disability and authentic representation is increasingly happening. But there are still real problems.

'I have to work twice as hard as my non-disabled colleagues to keep up with the long hours and punishing filming schedule. This often means waking up hours before the rest of the crew to factor in bowel management programmes, taking painkillers to keep going throughout the day, withholding food or water due to a lack of accessible toilets on location, staying in inaccessible places and even working in environments where disabled people aren't welcome. I often have to depend on a support worker to enable me to access the various places I go, which involves me being carried, lifted and manhandled. I'm usually one of the only disabled people in the crew too. "Another day, another ableist dickhead," I often find myself muttering under my breath.

'I remember when I first started working in TV, I found out that a non-disabled person doing the same job as me had been paid and I hadn't. The information had come to me by accident through a chance conversation. It made me feel like I was clearly valued less and that perhaps therefore my work was considered worthless. My heart sank. This validated my insecurities that I was only being used to tick a "disability" box and made me wonder how many other times I might have been duped into doing work for free when others around me weren't.'

The hostile environment that Morgan describes doesn't just make the industry difficult for disabled women to work in at times – it can make them leave it entirely. In 2023, presenter Melanie Sykes[12] – who was a staple of British television throughout the 2000s – spoke of how she quit the industry after receiving years of disturbing treatment as a woman with undiagnosed autism. As well as suffering repeated sexual harassment, Sykes disclosed that she struggled to work with the heightened sensitivities that can come with neurodivergence, such as using an earpiece needed for producers to talk to her. She turned to drinking as a way to cope.

Sykes isn't alone. A report by the regulatory body Ofcom in 2021[13] urged television and radio companies to focus on retaining women and disabled people due to the high numbers leaving the industry. The report predicted that if this exodus in broadcasting continues, the proportion of TV employees who are disabled and the number of female radio employees will actually fall by 2026 rather than grow. Barriers to people from minority groups staying in broadcasting were found to include disaffection with personal work experiences, feeling undervalued, and lack of support and sponsorship for underrepresented groups.

When broadcaster Fearne Cotton quit her flagship BBC Radio 1 show and later her job covering Radio 2 breakfast, few knew how the industry was affecting her mental health behind the scenes. Cotton, who has experienced anxiety and depression, had spent decades working successfully in high-profile radio and television roles. But after having increasingly frequent panic attacks in her early thirties, she decided to walk away. 'I think the panic attacks are a consequence of the job I've had for many years. Certain experiences where you're on the receiving end of harsh critique, trolling or abuse can take its toll and I found myself unable to cope with that pressure. At one point, I was having panic attacks several times throughout the day. I had to make some big decisions and one of them was to stop doing live radio until I felt I could cope with that pressure again. I didn't [speak to my bosses about my mental health]. I feared that it wouldn't go down well. My bosses [at Radio 1] were all older men at that time so I didn't feel comfortable approaching them with such personal issues.

'[When I was later covering for Zoe Ball on the Radio 2 breakfast show] it got to the point where I wouldn't sleep at all before the show so would turn up exhausted but wired. I would have these long, long panic attacks in bed, adrenaline surges and catastrophizing thoughts. If you go wrong on live radio there is no turning back. People are so unforgiving these days and I knew I wasn't strong enough to be cancelled or mocked if I got it wrong. It was terrifying leaving secure, celebrated jobs but I knew I needed change. I'm much happier doing the work I do today.

'I'm sure the TV industry is getting better but I don't feel there was any support while I was regularly on TV. I was lucky in the early days with two producers who nurtured the presenters on their kids' shows. I felt truly supported by them. Then I left the safe world of kids' TV and entered the tough domain of entertainment. It's pretty cut-throat. You're openly pitted against your peers, sacked without being told why, and given hell by the public if you put one foot wrong. It's a lot to deal with mentally. We know people still believe in the myth of celebrity but I'm not sure you can fully understand the darker side of it until you've been through it. I still can't face a lot of it and I've worked in this industry for twenty-six years.'

'TV has failed disabled people. Utterly and totally,' the writer Jack Thorne said in his MacTaggart Lecture – one of the most high-profile speeches in the media calendar – in 2021. 'Disability is the forgotten diversity, the one everyone leaves out of speeches. Gender, race, sexuality, all rightly get discussed at length. Disability gets relegated out. In conversations about representation, in action plans, and new-era planning, disability is confined to the corner, it remains an afterthought.'

Thorne – who himself has autism and whose writing credits include the *His Dark Materials* television adaptation and *Harry Potter and the Cursed Child* – saved particular criticism for the limited roles disabled actors are permitted to play. As he put it: 'The TV world is stacked against the telling of disabled stories with disabled talent.'

It's not hard to see what Thorne means. Roles for disabled female actors in Britain are few, and even more so if they won't accept the limited trope-heavy roles created for them. Disabled women are frequently characterized as one of a set stereotype: the previously healthy woman who tragically becomes disabled, subsequently going on to either live in misery or become magically healed by the next episode; the wise-cracking best friend of a non-disabled main character, never fleshed out or complex in her own right; if they are a main character, they are in an 'issue-driven' drama, typically about illness, poverty or death, where their disability must be the defining characteristic of their personality and life.

In contrast, disabled women on television or film are rarely depicted as thriving, sexual or powerful. Nor are they often portrayed as ordinary – a bored office worker or incompetent policewoman who just happens to have a disability. In fact, disabled characters are lucky if they get to talk at all. In 2022, the USC Annenberg study – which has tracked characters from minorities in each year's top-100 domestic films for the last fifteen years – found a minuscule 1.9 per cent of speaking characters in highest-grossing films had a visible disability.[14] Of those, most disabled characters were white and male. Only one character with a disability that year was LGBTQ+.

When there are disabled characters on-screen, there's not even a guarantee a disabled person will be playing them. Despite some pushback in recent years, it's still common for a non-disabled actor to be hired to play a disabled character – or to 'crip up', as it's often known. The scale of this is remarkable: one study found 95 per cent of characters with disabilities on television are played by non-disabled actors.[15]

Any disabled person who objects to this on social media is generally greeted with a mix of anger and condescension. 'It's called ACTING, love,' types FreeThinker26447. In contrast, there is very little backlash against the non-disabled actors taking these parts or the film-makers choosing to cast them. In fact, it's a great career move. Since 1947, out of fifty-nine Oscar nominations for disabled characters, twenty-seven have won an Academy Award. That's an almost 50 per cent success rate.[16] The number of winners who have had a real disability? Three.[17]

This practice across the industry deprives disabled actors of some of the few parts they could be seen as eligible to play, while suggesting disability is a costume to put on or physical act to mimic rather than a real characteristic, like race or sex. It also diminishes the sort of disabled stories we get to see, robbing popular culture of the authentic storytelling that comes from hiring creatives with lived experience in place of often hyper-sentimental 'inspiration porn'[18] made to tug at the heartstrings of the non-disabled audience.

Genevieve Barr knows this well. While non-disabled actors won applause for playing disabled characters, as a deaf actor and now a successful screenwriter, Barr struggled to get either disabled or non-disabled parts herself. 'When I started out as a deaf actor, I was reliably told I wouldn't be able to play any hearing parts and getting speaking roles would be very difficult. They said my voice "would have to be explained" and that I "could never pass for a hearing person". The audience "would have to work harder and it would confuse them", they said. Conversely, I didn't match up to what most directors and producers typically perceived as deaf in order to play a deaf character – usually somebody who used British Sign Language (BSL).

'I learned BSL to audition for deaf roles, which are few and far between, even now. I also went back to speech therapy for four years to work on my voice because it was viewed as my best chance of being perceived as "good enough" for the non-deaf parts. Was that discrimination? A barrier? Of course it was. I was told I didn't fit in. At the same time, I was told being deaf was the only thing they could see of me. It was confusing. And tiring. I wanted to feel like I was enough.'

As the star of the BBC's *The A Word* and *Ralph & Katie*, Sarah Gordy MBE is a rare example of a primetime actor with a learning disability. Gordy, who has Down's syndrome, has had to challenge people's preconceptions to get there. 'The attitude in the TV industry has changed a lot since I did my first professional TV job [in 2010]. My attitude was that I'm just another actor and they were surprised that I didn't slow down production. People have underestimated me. Sometimes they look at me and think I won't be able to remember lines or do my job. But I work hard and show them I can do it. Once they see my work, they're delighted. This in turn encourages them to go on to hire other actors with learning disabilities. There has been a lot of progress over the years. There are more people with learning disabilities on TV than there used to be, but there is room for a lot more in front of and behind the camera.

'All actors find it hard to get regular work. Many have to find other things to do. Only a few land recurring roles on big shows. I've had some great roles. [But] I can't say I had regular work. It is difficult for people with learning disabilities to get cast in certain roles. I wouldn't be cast as a lawyer or a scientist because I wouldn't be believable. However, in many other roles we can be uniquely brilliant. The writing is the most important thing. Real people are complicated. They have lots going on in their lives. A character with a learning disability should have more than their disability to be believable. We're all individuals. We're more than the label.'

For most actors, a prestigious award nomination marks the peak of their career opportunities. But when Ruth Madeley, who has spina bifida, was nominated for a BAFTA in 2016, she continued working in her day job at a charity, using her annual leave and weekends to audition for parts. As a disabled actor – even one at the top of her game – she feared there weren't enough roles for her to go full-time. 'Acting isn't particularly stable work to begin with [but] the distinct lack of opportunity for disabled artists [means] it becomes even harder to carve out a career. I never thought it would be sustainable and something I could do for a living long-term.'

Madeley is now flourishing as an in-demand actor but says she's still treated differently because of her disability. 'I often feel like I have to work harder than anyone else in the room as a disabled actress. You have to prove you can play any role regardless of disability and that can be tough mentally. My role in *Years and Years* wasn't originally intended to be a wheelchair user but it was changed after my audition, which was an incredible experience. It's definitely becoming more of a conversation now, having disabled actors audition for all roles, but I wouldn't say it's common practice. Disability representation is incredibly far behind where it needs to be.

'I've had to have some really tough conversations with producers about access, like when I've been on a set and accessible toilets haven't been provided. I've had props left on the seat of my wheelchair when I've been sat out of it, as if it's a prop rather than my personal disability aid. At the start of my career I found it really hard to point out any access issues. I never wanted to rock the boat or "cause a problem". I'm definitely more confident now as I know I have a responsibility for the actors coming into the industry after me. But that doesn't mean the conversations get any easier.'

These conversations are hard but they are thankfully increasingly happening – not only prompted by actors themselves but also the execs at the top of the industry. In 2022, the TV Access Project (TAP) – a coalition of ten of the UK's biggest broadcasters and streamers – was formed with the aim of delivering real improvements in access for disabled talent across the television industry. In the coming years, the coalition hopes to achieve goals including adequate funding for access costs, more disabled people in senior decision-making roles, and accountability for broadcasters and streamers to achieve disability inclusion.

Genevieve Barr – who helped set up the coalition after her own experiences – believes progress is already being made. 'It's an industry that's changing, albeit slowly. There's increasingly a watchful gaze on who writes these stories, accurate casting, and the hiring of access consultants from broadcasters and commissioners. Disabled people have been invisible on our screens since time began and creating an end product where accurate, nuanced portrayals of disabled lives regularly reach the millions of audiences is something that needs a lot of effort from a lot of people. Access is the thing that needs to be addressed before good representation can become commonplace. Film and television sets are made of wood and wires and honeywagons with steps, toilets with narrow doors, a thirteen-hour day on-set. It's shocking how inaccessible it is. In 2021, we ran a survey of seventy-two studios and facilities, and found only one accessible toilet available for hire across the UK.[19]

'Then there's the culture on sets. People are usually hired only a few weeks before production starts and don't know another person on-set. This can be scary as a new person trying to break into the industry and also difficult to maintain relationships to stay there. It can be hard to ask for help, but really the issue is we shouldn't have to. Disabled people should be able to come in on their first day, do their job and know who to talk to if something's needed. But the industry isn't set up that way. Right now, our coalition effort – the TV Access Project – is bringing together broadcasters, streamers, disabled professionals and others to find a standardized approach to try and come up with solutions. We're normalizing access coordinators – a production role for access. And there's more and more to come. Our collective goal for TAP is that by 2030, the industry is fully accessible to all disabled people. There's a lot we can do. Good things. I'm hopeful that we're in a different gear than we were.'

As an actor with Ehlers–Danlos syndrome, Jameela Jamil is already seeing that change. 'I've definitely crafted my career around my health. You have to with a condition like mine. I demand less time in hair and make-up – I refuse to come in earlier than the men! – because it's hard to sleep because of pain, so I need extra rest. I don't fly a lot because I have very delicate eardrums that love to burst. I tell people I will never be toned, because exercise hurts and I can't be arsed. I'm a comedian not an Olympian. I will always look and feel like a long memory-foam mattress.

'I'm very unapologetic about turning down action films and TV shows; no fame or money is worth compromising my health and peace. [When I took on the Marvel She-Hulk job] I didn't know it was an action role when I signed the deal. Everything is always top secret with these shows! But once I found out, after a year and a half in lockdown [during the pandemic], I felt like setting some new challenges for myself . . . so I decided to jump in and really learn the stunts and the martial arts myself. They were extremely mindful about my wellbeing. They paid for a trainer who's experienced with my disability and an amazing stunts team, as well as access to physiotherapy when the inevitable dislocations came knocking. I ended up doing 90 per cent of my own stunts, and while it wasn't easy, I'm really excited I got to learn this new side to my body, and to be able to see that this industry doesn't always have to treat people like a burden. Everyone should take notes.'

'She looks tired'

When I was young, we had 'Blair's Babes'. In the late 90s, the election of Tony Blair's Labour government brought a record number of female MPs into Parliament and, with it, a genuine sense of progress for women in politics – albeit with a depressingly sexist moniker from parts of the media. Since then, female representation has continued to grow: while we're still a way off a 50:50 gender split of MPs, women now make up 40 per cent of the House of Commons.[20] If you're a disabled woman, though, that picture is far less optimistic. Disabled people barely make up 1 per cent of the House of Commons[21] – the equivalent of a handful out of 650 seats. If we were just counting disabled women MPs, I wouldn't need much more than my thumbs.

So, what's keeping disabled women out of political office? Recent years have seen headlines rightly highlighting how Westminster can be a hostile environment for women, from accusations of sexual harassment to inadequate childcare facilities.[22] What's rarely discussed, though, is how a political career can be hostile to disabled people too. Research for the Government Equalities Office by the University of London and the University of Strathclyde in 2021[23] found disabled people face a number of barriers when participating in party politics: from poor accessibility of venues, financial barriers, inaccessible formatting of materials, to bureaucratic processes which make it harder to get reasonable adjustments (which all disabled people are legally entitled to).

The unique set-up of Parliament means becoming an MP can be particularly out of reach. If a disabled MP doesn't have the access arrangements they need in the office, there's no HR department to go to for help. If a backbencher is struggling with fatigue, they still have to drag themselves to the lobby for a midnight vote. This can be even harder for the few disabled women in senior positions, such as members of government. In 2023, Levelling Up Minister Dehenna Davison resigned from her cabinet role due to chronic migraines.[24] The thirty-year-old – thought to be a rising star of the Conservative Party at the time – said it was 'difficult, if not impossible to keep up with the demands of ministerial life' alongside her condition.

As the first ever full-time wheelchair user in the House of Commons, Dame Anne Begg knows all too well the obstacles of being a disabled woman in politics. Elected as part of the record-breaking new cohort of female MPs in 1997, 'every effort' was made to allow her access to the nineteenth-century Chamber – but Begg remembers the many difficulties too. 'The Palace of Westminster is an old building and the width of individual doors was so variable. On one occasion I turned up for a meeting with Robin Cook – the then Foreign Secretary – and found I couldn't get into his office.

'I quickly learned to contact the places I was going to beforehand to ensure the location was accessible. Voting was also a problem. The Yes and No voting lobbies each had three doors, and depending on the letter of the alphabet that your name began with, you were supposed to go through the correct door. I could only get through one of these doors so I had to shout over to my own teller to record my vote. I insisted I wanted to record my own individual vote rather than by proxy. At first, I couldn't access a toilet near my office so every time I needed to go, I had to trek far away. In the end, they installed an accessible toilet for me near my office. Outside Parliament, travel by train was full of difficulties. On one Select Committee visit I was "allocated" to the guard's van. The rest of the committee didn't want me to sit there on my own so they all joined me in the guard's van for the journey.'

Baroness Emma Nicholson, who was born deaf, has experienced life as a disabled politician across multiple different offices of state over the years. As a Conservative and later Liberal Democrat MP in the 1980s and 1990s, a member of the Council of Europe, and now a life peer in the House of Lords, Nicholson has often been the only deaf person in the room. 'The House of Commons was a great place in which to be profoundly deaf. Everyone shouts so inevitably no one can hear. I was normal! And since people could not hear each other they asked all of the time, "What did so and so say?" I felt one of the crowd. And it's a small chamber so even with my weak eyesight I could sometimes lip-read across the floor. Neil Kinnock had a particularly easy face. When I was later a member of the Council of Europe, they carefully analysed what I needed and installed special equipment in the Chamber at my seat – a headset cleverly plugged into the electronic system – and a staff member behind me. It transformed my work. During my decade in the European Parliament, the officials provided headphones and a translator. That gave me the best chance ever of fully joining in the debates.

'The first time I encountered prejudice on my deafness was in the House of Lords, which was a big and highly unwelcome shock. The prejudice has been constant and ongoing.

I've experienced some really odd behaviour, like "Did your hearing aids cause the lights in the Chamber to go out?" comments. If I quietly ask a colleague what someone has said, I get slapped down for disturbance in the Chamber. Once, even by letter from the Lord Speaker. I'm not the only peer to feel that [some colleagues] have a sense of disbelief that your disability is real, not fake.

'There's a view that the only protected characteristics to note in politics are those connected with sex and gender. This became very clear when we were all forced to attend diversity training sessions but there was no mention of disability. I asked about it but there was no answer given. I wrote the question on the form and received no reply. I wrote a letter and it was ignored. The Lords now has three diversity officers but no disability officer or discussion or help. We're one in five of the population, so why are we being ignored?'

As one of the new generation of disabled MPs, Marsha de Cordova has experienced first-hand the progress that's been made to parliamentary access in the decades since Begg and Nicholson's time in office. Since her election in 2017 for the Labour Party, de Cordova, who is registered blind, has been able to reach the heights of the shadow cabinet as Shadow Minister for Women and Equality. But day-to-day, she still faces dangerously poor disability access. 'Having the Palace of Westminster as my workplace is quite something, but it's far from fully accessible to me. It has poor lighting, a lack of colour contrasting, no delineation on steps and not enough accessible lifts. I've fallen down steps a few times. I avoided being seriously injured but it did cause slight bruising. Fortunately, colleagues were on hand to help as well as the doorkeepers. It was very upsetting. I have a big fear of steps.

'The voting machines aren't accessible so it is difficult to be certain that my vote has been registered. I have to wait to hear the bleep, but this can be difficult as the division lobbies are busy and can be noisy. [There is no other] option available for me to cast my vote. As a Black disabled woman, I face indirect forms of prejudice and stereotyping on two levels. I've been mistaken for a fellow Black female MP. I constantly have to ask for documents to be in accessible format or for other provisions to be in place because people don't realize or believe that I'm partially sighted blind, just because I don't use a physical aid to help me move around.

'There has been some progress over the years. Following my calls, there have been some changes made to the parliamentary estate including tactile markings on some steps and some fluorescent markings on glass doors . . . but there needs to be collective responsibility. It's not right that change in Parliament only happens once disabled politicians call for it.'

As de Cordova has worryingly found, many of the barriers facing disabled MPs are physical: from inaccessible voting machines to dangerously lit stairways. But we also know some of the barriers are cultural – or to put it another way, the attitude that says disabled people don't belong in politics (so why bother making it accessible?). For an insight into this, look how world leaders are treated the moment they show signs of disability. At over eighty years old, it became the norm for US President Joe Biden – who has severe spinal arthritis – to have his health monitored by the media and public. In 2024, Biden chose not to run for a second term after a series of gaffs led to intense questions about his mental capacity, but it's notable that even minor signs of physical disability had long been used as evidence he was not fit for office: from him slipping as he got on to Air Force One[25] to journalists demanding he 'explain his slow walk'.[26] Meanwhile, the late Queen Elizabeth may have never had to worry about seeking re-election but as a Head of State she nonetheless felt the need to not 'look disabled' in public. Insiders reported that the Queen insisted on a 'military-style exercise' during her Platinum Jubilee in 2023[27] to avoid being photographed using a wheelchair. Eighty years after Franklin D. Roosevelt used a cloak to hide his wheelchair from the electorate,[28] power is still seen as incompatible with disability. As much as I would like to say otherwise, I simply cannot imagine a prime minister standing outside Downing Street with a white cane or hearing aid. There is a reason why a headline reading 'She looks tired' is known as the end of a woman's political career.[29]

These prejudices do not just perpetuate the idea that people with health conditions should not be in politics – they normalize a relentless work culture that criticizes and doubts any politician showing signs of 'weakness'. Being an MP is a notoriously brutal career. Unlike other jobs, in the House of Commons there's no working-from-home option, nor a chance to go part-time or job-share. This fast pace is even more alienating when you consider the emotional toll the job can take, from the rise of abuse towards MPs on social media in recent years (particularly towards women of colour)[30] to the long hours away from family. In 2023, former Deputy Prime Minister Thērēse Coffey – who has not got a disclosed disability – reported that she became so ill during her time in government that she 'nearly died'.[31] 'I was in hospital for a month with some of the stresses that happen with ministerial life,' she said. 'I worked myself into the ground.' If this is happening to MPs without pre-existing health conditions, it's not hard to imagine what the strain might be on those with one. It is not as if it's straightforward for an MP to take time off when the workload gets too much. Many are expected to simply 'power through' physical or mental health problems, no matter the consequences.

When Nadia Whittome MP took time off for PTSD in 2021, she found herself tackling the House of Commons' outdated traditions on sick leave as well as prejudice around mental health. 'For a few months, my symptoms had been getting worse [and] having a severe impact on my life. Speaking to my doctor, it became clear that in order to get better I needed to make the time and space for my recovery that just doesn't exist when you're regularly working seven days a week, so that meant taking time off. On my doctor's advice, I took the decision to take a [three-month] leave of absence from my MP duties. That time off work was invaluable – it allowed me to get the kind of treatment I needed to help reduce my symptoms.

'I felt guilty about stepping back from a role that I felt so privileged to hold and that so many people had entrusted me with. I received a lot of support from my Labour colleagues, and from MPs in other parties, [while the] front-bench and the whips backed my decision. I was also overwhelmed by the support from constituents and from people across the country who had experience of PTSD or of needing to take time off for their mental health.

'But there was a backlash too, primarily on social media and right-wing blog sites. There were comments claiming that I didn't really have PTSD because I was young and I'd never been in a war, or that this proved that I wasn't up to the job of being an MP. There was also a lot of speculation, including in the national press, about what might have caused my PTSD. I avoided reading comments on social media. It's clear that the system is not set up for MPs to be able to take a leave of absence. While my office continued to do casework for constituents, there were some things that just couldn't happen while I was away, such as submitting questions to ministers. Because of the pandemic, voting by proxy was allowed at the time so I continued to vote, but if I took a leave of absence now, that wouldn't be possible.'

It isn't just that doing the job of an MP can be harder if you're disabled – it can be tough to even get elected in the first place. The same research by the University of London and the University of Strathclyde[32] discovered a range of obstacles for disabled candidates during their election campaigns. This included a lack of accessible transport, inaccessible buildings and the inaccessibility of hustings (particularly for neurodivergent or Deaf candidates). Some disabled people also reported facing heightened scrutiny and negative attitudes that they weren't 'up to the job' because of their disability. It echoes what Dame Begg told me: 'I remember once when campaigning for the 1997 election, one future constituent said he wouldn't vote for me. He didn't believe that I would manage to do my duties as an MP by being able to attend the House of Commons.'

One of the best ways to counter this sort of prejudice is for disabled candidates to meet voters, but they are often physically excluded from campaigning. Interviewees in the University of London research reported that prospective disabled MPs had been prevented from attending local party meetings or campaign events due to lack of access, such as fundraising events being booked in pubs with no lifts. One interviewee said they were unable to attend local party meetings since being told that an accessible toilet would cost too much, while an MP said that their party 'just didn't have any money' to spend on induction loops in order to make meetings accessible for Deaf people. As a result, it's often the disabled candidates themselves who are left to cover the extra costs, be it hiring their own British Sign Language interpreter, printing material in accessible formats, or paying for taxis to get around. Notably, the Access to Elected Office Fund once covered disability-related costs for parliamentary and other elections, but it was closed by the Conservative government in 2015.[33]*

As a cross-bench member of the House of Lords, Baroness Jane Campbell – who uses a wheelchair and a BiPAP to help her breathe – has had to fight to gain adjustments to Parliament's archaic rules that work for her disability. But as a politician who was appointed rather than elected, Campbell says she – and other disabled people like her – would never have been able to withstand the demanding election process needed to be an MP. 'When I arrived, there wasn't even a fully accessible changing-table bathroom that I could use. However, with my involvement we made some pretty significant alterations both to my office and nearby accessible toilet. Where it was more of a

---

* In response to a legal case brought by three disabled politicians, the government was forced to set up a temporary, partial replacement, the EnAble Fund, but that ran out in 2019, and it was not open to disabled candidates standing in the general election.

struggle was when I made a request to bring a PA [personal assistant] into the Debating Chamber. It meant overturning a parliamentary rule that "no commoner must cross the bar into the Chamber, only ennobled Peers, doorkeepers and clerks to the Chamber"! It took me two years to overturn the ruling. Some Members were reluctant to make changes to any of the Lords' ceremonies and protocols, which were preventing my equal participation in my parliamentary role. I needed a lot of confidence and resilience during this time.

'Some of the way in which we work would not suit disabled people who might have medical conditions which cause fatigue, or concentration issues. The meetings are often lengthy and go late into the evening. There is little leeway in terms of the timetable and virtually no breaks in long debates. Lunch hours and a dinner break if you're lucky. I would never have the stamina or physical capability to be an elected member of Parliament in the House of Commons. I think the route to becoming an elected member is gruelling and there are still a lot of discriminatory attitudes which get in the way of the process. There remains a significant lack of representation from disabled people and very little evidence of it improving.'

This isn't just detrimental for those disabled women who dream of going into politics – it damages wider society too. The wave of government policies that have disproportionately harmed disabled people in recent years – from benefit cuts, to the underfunding of social care and the NHS – shows starkly the consequences of poor disability representation. When a politician has never had to apply for disability benefits themselves, it's much easier to vote to reduce them. That isn't to say that simply having more disabled MPs would guarantee change. Just as Liz Truss becoming prime minister did nothing to help women's day-to-day lives, more disabled MPs will mean little if they work against the disabled community's interests. But it is to say that having disabled people in the room inevitably improves the chances of our needs being addressed.

Besides, there is something nigglingly perverse about a group of non-disabled people making decisions that affect millions of disabled people's lives – and a culture that says this is perfectly OK. Nowadays, if a committee on women's reproductive health was run solely by men, social media would rightly be filled with outrage – but when non-disabled MPs legislate about disability issues, it's somehow widely seen as acceptable. In many ways, disabled people being governed solely by non-disabled politicians is the ultimate example of the infantilizing attitudes towards disability that we've seen throughout this book. If disabled women are ever going to be fully respected and valued, we must surely reach the point where we are seen as credible leaders and decision-makers in our own right. As the old disability rights slogan goes: 'Nothing about us, without us.'

Britain's missing model

In the summer of 2023,[34] British model Sian Green-Lord noticed something odd. A photograph she had posted on Instagram of herself in a swimsuit wearing a prosthetic leg had ended up in a summer campaign by the Spanish government. Except it wasn't quite her. Green-Lord's image had been used – but they had airbrushed out her prosthesis.

'I don't even know how to even explain the amount of anger that I'm feeling right now . . . I'm literally shaking, I'm so angry,' she said[35] to media outlets at the time. 'It's one thing using my image without my permission, but it's another thing editing my body, my body with my prosthetic leg . . . I don't even know what to say but it's beyond wrong.'

In an ironic twist, the doctored image was used as part of a body-positivity promotion called 'Summer is ours too' – run by Spain's equality ministry – 'as a response to fatphobia, hatred and the questioning of non-normative bodies'. All bodies are welcome (just not those gross disabled ones).

I would like to say I was shocked by this, but then I would be lying. From the first time I bought a teen magazine with my pocket money, I learned very quickly that the world did not want to gaze at girls who looked like me. It was funny, really, how I barely noticed something that would stay with me for decades. There was no big realization, no date on the calendar I can mark out as the day it hit me. I understood implicitly that beautiful spaces were not supposed to be for disabled women and I understood without anyone ever saying it out loud. As I have grown older, that silent message has not been challenged. Whether it is advertising campaigns, the covers of magazines, or on the runway, it is still the norm for women to scan the latest trends and not see a single disabled model staring back at us.

Disability is in many ways the last taboo in fashion. While the representation of black women, trans women and other minorities has thankfully increased in the industry in recent years, women with disabilities – especially visible disabilities – are still incredibly rare, despite being the largest minority in the world. The scale of this is ludicrous. One recent study found that disabled people make up just 0.02 per cent of models featured in fashion campaigns.[36] Things are little better when we consider the industry as a whole. A 2024 census of the UK fashion industry by the British Fashion Council (BFC)[37] showed that of the 1,529 survey participants, only 6 per cent identified as disabled.

Laura Winson, the founder of Zebedee Talent, an agency representing models with disabilities and visible differences, says: 'Disability is definitely lagging behind other diverse characteristics, such as race and curve models. You only have to look at all the Fashion Weeks across the world to see that. You can count on one hand the number of disabled people on the runway. There are practical barriers in front of disabled models, anything from audition rooms not being wheelchair accessible to designers being unwilling to spend resources on a sign language interpreter. But the biggest issue is that casting directors simply aren't considering disabled people. We've worked with excellent high-end brands, but overall there's still reluctance to hire disabled models. We constantly reach out to brands. We get little to no response.'

In some ways, none of this is surprising. The fashion industry is not well known for its forward-thinking approach to women's bodies. Disability does not fit easily in a professional culture that demands physical perfection (and generally defines perfection as being incredibly thin), just as disabled women will struggle to represent aspirational beauty in a society that too often equates disability and sickness with ugliness and sadness. When nondisabled models are still airbrushed to be 'acceptable', those with scars and canes are hardly going to be widely seen as palatable.

As the winner of the BBC's *Britain's Missing Top Model* in 2008, Kelly Knox became one of the first visibly disabled models to get a foothold in the industry. Knox, who was born without a left forearm, has since graced the cover of *Grazia* and fronted brand campaigns including Primark but it's not always been easy. 'Back in 2008, when I first took part in the show, there were zero disabled models working in the fashion industry. We were shown a video of a model at Fashion Week and she said, "Fashion Week would rather burn down than see a disabled person on the runway." I had something to prove – I wanted to show that disabled people are not only worthy of representation, but are cool, hot, fashionable and can do it as well as any other "able-bodied" model.

'I was signed to a major agency at the time but I was the only disabled model and probably the only size-12 model. I felt like I needed to grow an arm and lose weight. I couldn't possibly have one hand *and* be a size 12. At the beginning, I was told I'd get more work if I wore a prosthetic arm. They meant, if I looked "normal". I refused. I'm not here to be normalized. I'm here to stand out in my full glory. I remember receiving a nasty comment from a troll on one of my pictures. They said, "Grow an arm you fucking ugly disabled bitch." It was funny, really, because I was shooting Savage Fenty lingerie at the Ritz. It didn't bother me but it shows how people see us: below them.

'Within six months, the agency went into liquidation. It was horrendous. They stopped responding to my emails and calls. I was left to navigate this strange industry without representation. I felt like I was left in the gutter. My first proper agency signing was years later in 2017. There has been change since I started but not enough. Disabled people are still not used regularly enough in campaigns. At the beginning of my career, it did feel like tokenism. Now, there are lots of incredible brands who believe in the power of diversity and book models like myself for the right reasons. I'm happy to see lots of disabled people representing themselves on social media, helping to challenge perceptions and break barriers. There's still a hell of a lot of work to do.'

Fifteen years on from when Knox began her career, the fashion industry has certainly made some strides to represent disability. As we saw in the chapter on body image, adaptive clothing – though limited – is slowly becoming more mainstream as more brands and stores learn to be accessible to disabled shoppers. When it comes to the faces of the industry, there has also been some progress (even if that progress lags behind other diverse groups). Adwoa Aboah, who has spoken openly about her depression, and Bella Hadid, who has Lyme disease, are some of the most high-profile models working today. It is easier, of course, for the industry to accept models whose disabilities are hidden – no designer has to worry that Aboah or Hadid 'look disabled' when they put them on the runway or challenge any preconceptions by hiring them – but there have slowly been some gains for visible disabilities too. In 2023, British *Glamour* put three disabled women on its digital cover for its annual 'self-love' issue: from influencers who use electric wheelchairs, to a ventilator user.[38] In the same year, British *Vogue*[39] launched its first ever 'disability issue', in which it featured a range of visibly disabled women as cover stars.

Ellie Goldstein, who has Down's syndrome, was one of the models chosen for British *Vogue*'s iconic edition. It was the latest in a string of covers for her – Goldstein has also appeared on the front of *Glamour* and *Elle* – as well as brand campaigns. In 2020, Goldstein became the first model with a disability to represent Gucci. 'It was amazing when I got the Gucci beauty campaign. I couldn't believe it. I felt so lucky and honoured to represent other people with disabilities. I was so glad that I could show the world nothing would hold me back from my dreams. The response was amazing. On Instagram, it was Gucci's most liked picture, with just under a million likes and most comments – over six thousand. Ninety-five per cent of the comments were positive. There were a couple of stupid replies, like "Gucci is going downhill." But it didn't bother me. I've never felt [discriminated against] on any shoot or interview. My mum always comes to shoots with me, and if she can't, my mum's friend takes me. She really enjoys seeing how the shoot works. If there are stairs [to get around a venue], I take it slow. I think the industry is getting better with representation but it still has a long way to go. I think brands are a bit scared still to use models that look different.'

As founder of Tilting the Lens – an agency which consults with fashion brands on accessibility – Sinéad Burke is working to challenge that fear. Burke, who has the short limb condition achondroplasia, became invested in fashion as a teenager to 'challenge the assumptions about me and my body' and has since become one of the most visible figures making change in the industry. 'For me, attending the Met Gala [in 2019] was a key moment. Due to the red carpet taking place on a flight of stairs, physically disabled people were and are so often excluded. I felt very proud to attend, particularly as it ignited my tenure on Gucci's Global Equity Board, but even more, thinking about the young people who look like me, who might for the first time know that it was possible for them too. I used a foot-stool to stand on and Anna Wintour arranged for it to be covered in the same fabric as the carpet. Chic!

'I often find myself wondering if this increased visibility changed the fashion industry, or if it just changed it for me? There have definitely been measurable, collective shifts: Aaron Rose Philip on the runway for Moschino and Collina Strada; Ellie Goldstein in a Gucci beauty campaign; and Chella Man for Calvin Klein and Nike. But has it become easier for disabled people to work in the fashion industry, to study design, to have a part-time job in retail or to buy garments that fit? For long-term inclusive change to happen, leaders within the organizations have to get behind this work. From HR leads, marketing executives, store planning experts, museum curators, storytellers, digital innovators, design teams, creative directors and CEOs.'

'No one wants to watch a musician who looks like that'

In the summer of 2023, metre-high flags colouring the sky, Lewis Capaldi took to the stage at Glastonbury. Capaldi – who has Tourette's syndrome and anxiety – gave a stellar performance, but as the set went on, his tics visibly increased. As he struggled with his symptoms, Capaldi admitted to the crowd that he was losing his voice. 'I just need you all to sing with me as loud as you can, if that's OK?' he asked. In an exchange that went viral,[40] Capaldi's fans didn't let him down. By the end of the set, the audience had taken over completely, chanting his lyrics back to him. Capaldi simply stood on the stage taking it in: a sea of smiling faces stretched as far as the eye could see, a hundred thousand voices singing in unison.

It was a genuinely moving moment of disability acceptance, made all the more so because of how unusual that is. It isn't simply that it's rare to see disabled musicians being accepted – it's rare to see disabled musicians full stop. Scan the Top 40 chart or Spotify 'most played' and you will struggle to find more than a handful of artists with a disclosed disability – or often, any at all. There are a few well-known exceptions. Like Capaldi, Billie Eilish has Tourette's syndrome. Justin Bieber has been diagnosed with Ramsay Hunt syndrome, which paralysed one side of his face, while Chappell Roan has bipolar.[41] Lady Gaga, meanwhile, has the chronic pain condition fibromyalgia. And yet these are markedly sparse examples, most of whom developed a disability when their career and fanbase was already well established. Overall, the music industry has an astonishing deficit in promoting disabled talent, particularly when it comes to representation on commercial or major record labels. At this point of the chapter, I would like to include statistics about the number of disabled artists fronting festivals or winning major industry awards but there is no information available. Nowadays, each year there is, rightly, pushback on the lack of female headliners at UK festivals or the male dominance of the BRIT Awards shortlist. If you're a disabled woman in music, no one even bothers counting.

Suzanne Bull MBE, founder of music and live-events charity Attitude is Everything, who herself uses a wheelchair, says there are many reasons for this underrepresentation. 'We have some household names of bands and solo artists now who are openly disabled. But there's still not enough, particularly signed to mainstream record companies or getting headline spots. I remember one promoter sharing a major festival line-up with me with all the non-disabled artists taken out and unsurprisingly the line-up was completely blank. At the same time, it's really hard to know the true number because many artists who are disabled are afraid to identify as such, especially because there's pressure from the labels and managers not to. There's a certain kind of disabled artist who is accepted. If you can hide your impairment, you're encouraged to do so. If you're disabled but don't look it, that's acceptable. If your disability doesn't come with any perceived complications, that means you're easier and cheaper to work with.

'There's a myriad of barriers for disabled musicians, from the obvious physical barriers to accessing recording studios and rehearsal spaces, or touring being exhausting, to grass-roots venues not being accessible for building audiences. If disabled artists don't have their access arrangements met, it's highly unlikely they'll be able to work at their best. When I was in a band years ago, I once had to play on the floor in my wheelchair while the rest of the band played on the stage behind me. Then there's issues such as whether a disabled person is deemed capable enough to take up music at school by teachers in the first place. Barriers in the music industry for disabled people are also based on selling sex and glamour. Even as recently as two years ago, one of our female disabled artists was dropped by her management because she had to start using a disability aid. Her management said, "No one will want to look at anyone like that!"'

After winning *The Voice UK* in 2013, overnight Andrea Begley became one of the only mainstream disabled musicians in the country. Begley, who is visually impaired, was subsequently signed to the label Capitol Records and scored a Top 10 with her debut album. But after only a year, her contract was suspended. 'The industry is a tough business.

Despite my initial chart success, I was let go by my label. I have no doubt that I've been overlooked and undermined due to my disability on many occasions but discrimination is rarely done "to your face", it's usually subtle and unspoken. I received criticism from the public and the media who saw my win as nothing more than a victory for the sympathy vote. Being disabled in public life still has a sense of oddity about it. I don't recall meeting many, if any, disabled artists who worked full-time in the music business, and definitely not any disabled artists who were signed to the main record companies. After my contract ended, I went back to work as a civil servant and release music independently now.

'I think most people would seriously struggle to name a Top 10 of disabled people who are prevalent in the music business and that's not because there aren't extremely talented disabled artists out there. There are many practical barriers in the music industry for disabled musicians. The key one for me is driving. To get to a gig with my equipment, I have to rely a lot on family and friends. I'll need to win the lottery for a chauffeur. Even basic equipment like guitar tuners, speakers and loop pedals are all designed for non-disabled artists. Social media has definitely revolutionized access to wider audiences. You can upload a video on TikTok or YouTube and reach across the globe in a way you never could before. But independently taking videos or pictures and editing them proves inaccessible a lot of the time for me. It's not the first time I've uploaded a picture of my foot instead of me playing at a gig, but at least it keeps my fans entertained.' Begley is far from alone in experiencing these practical barriers. Research by Attitude is Everything in 2019[42] found disabled musicians face career-damaging obstacles when seeking to rehearse, record and play live. As many as half of the disabled artists surveyed had encountered access barriers to rehearsal spaces. Some 70 per cent said they have withheld details of their health condition or disability due to worries it would negatively impact relationships with promoters, venues or festivals. Of those playing live, two in three said they have compromised their health or wellbeing to perform. This discrimination can be even worse for disabled musicians of colour. A separate survey by Attitude is Everything and Black Lives Matter in Music in 2023[43] found 74 per cent of black disabled music creators felt there are specific barriers to success in the industry because of their race or ethnicity compared to 58 per cent of black non-disabled creators who felt the same way.

Just like we've seen in other chapters on healthcare or careers, barriers for disabled people to flourish in the music industry don't have to be physical – they can be rooted in cultural prejudice too. If a festival booker thinks disabled people are less capable than their non-disabled peers, they'll naturally doubt a musician with a disability can handle a headline slot. If a magazine editor believes disability is unsexy and off-putting to fans, they'll be less likely to pick a visibly disabled artist for that coveted front cover. When

Lewis Capaldi performed at Glastonbury, it was notable that, amongst the positive reactions, some social media users were openly uncomfortable with seeing his tics. 'If he's doing that, he shouldn't be on-stage' was a common response, as if to say: 'You can be disabled if you must but please don't do it where I have to see.' This discomfort – or worse, revulsion – at disability is only encouraged by parts of the media who perpetuate the idea it is quite literally headline news if a musician is spotted showing signs of a health condition. When Sam Smith was photo-graphed[44] wearing a leg brace and using a cane in 2024, the press filled column inches with their 'concern' for the singer while pawing over the possible causes. The same treatment has been levelled at many artists over the years, from Elton John, with his walking stick,[45] to Jessie J and her broken ankle.[46] The message is twofold: disability is an oddity worthy of gossip, and famous singers – idealized as aspirational, wealthy and attractive – should hide behind closed doors rather than commit the sin of being 'seen disabled' in public.

As frontwoman of the indie band Idealistics, Ali Hirsz has been played on BBC 6 Music and Radio X as well as being featured in the *NME*. But Hirsz – who has a con-nective tissue condition and uses a feeding tube – says dis-crimination in the industry over her visible disability has repeatedly stalled the band's opportunities to succeed com-mercially. 'Less than a year after forming, we were playing regular venues and in talks with a few small labels and management companies. Within a month of my tube being fitted we'd been told we couldn't play any of the venues any more unless we had a reputable promoter with other bands playing on the same night because my feeding tube would "deter crowds" as it wasn't "easy on the eyes". Managers said it would be much harder to push us as a band now and labels said that they'd be taking a gamble on a young band that will probably dissolve anyway because I was so poorly. Most of these discussions were over the phone. Every time I asked for something in writing everyone refused. That makes it harder to fight.

'It was also really hard to find promoters who would work with us because of my feeding tube. We had a major promoter tell us straight up they would never put our band on, no matter how successful we got, because of my feeding tube. They didn't think they would make ticket sales. Our last booking agent was pretty good until I had to cancel a show in London due to being hospitalized with sepsis and a heart infection. I received nasty phone calls while in my hospital bed, demanding proof from consultants. Then they refused calls and emails. They still owe us money from one of the shows.

'I've had members of management and promotion companies within the industry call me ableist slurs, such as "cripple". I thought perhaps they didn't realize and did my best to politely point out that they were not words to be used. They found it incredibly funny and responded with "snowflake". I've also struggled with other artists. I've had [them] tell me I had no right to take opportunities from others who could "use it to its full potential". One artist I really respected told me that if I wanted to get anywhere, I couldn't show my weaknesses. I remember being so shocked that my disability was viewed as a weakness. It really awakened me to the industry.'

When Victoria Canal, who has a lower limb amputation, signed a recording deal with Parlophone Records in 2022, she became one of the few visibly disabled women in the industry to be represented by a mainstream record label. But Canal – who guest-starred for Coldplay at their Glastonbury headline show in 2024 – says she still experiences prejudice about her disability. 'The media has historically talked about me differently – such as using my disability in the headline with no mention of my name, or hardly talking about the music in interviews and focusing on the "inspiration porn" angle of it all. [When Canal first worked with Coldplay's frontman, the headlines ran: 'Chris Martin plays with pianist with one hand.']47 But I feel like the discrimination is mostly social. Something I've experienced a few times is when an artist treats me relatively shitty until they're made aware of what I'm up to and who I am. Suddenly, I'm not the weird girl with one arm bothering them any more – they want to write with me, they want to know me. That's a really jarring feeling that I've felt tenfold. It's weird to say that out loud, I've never really talked about that before. But I really feel it.

'I feel like there's this super "performative diversity" thing happening within corporate marketing that's just desperately trying to catch up with where society is going in terms of representation and awareness. I definitely know why I'm being hired for certain things. It's no secret I tick a box. Or many boxes – I am queer, Latina, and disabled, after all. It takes a lot of routinely convincing myself that it's not just my labels that have gotten me to this place in my career.'

The 'performative diversity' Canal points to is certainly an increasing issue in creative industries: superficial tokenism that notices society's push towards inclusion and wants to piggyback on to it without actually doing anything useful. I can't help but think every company who puts out a social media post on World Mental Health Day should be legally required to publish how many people they've hired with mental health conditions. Real diversity in the music industry – like change anywhere – is harder, slower, and often starts behind closed doors. It is the work of disabled-led organizations such as Attitude is Everything and Drake Music,[48] the national arts charity that uses technology to make music more accessible. It is Ticketmaster announcing in 2023 it would at last enable disabled gig-goers to book online 'like anyone else'[49] rather than queuing on premium-rate phone lines for hours.

I feel hope whenever I see artists being open about their health conditions. Mercury Prize winner Arlo Parks has spoken frankly about her depression and wrote her hit single 'Black Dog' about her experience.[50] Legendary singer Cēline Dion[51] went public with her diagnosis of 'stiff person syndrome', a neurological disease that leads to severe muscle spasms. Elsewhere, Lady Gaga has spoken about her experience with chronic pain and what she describes as psychotic breaks. 'At some point, I had to tell people,' she said to Oprah Winfrey in 2020.[52] 'I can't live a lie, I'm an authentic person, and here I am, I'm perfectly imperfect, and we all are. We all have our things that we go through. I felt like, "Why shouldn't I share this when I share all of myself with the world all the time?"'

No disabled artist is under any obligation to disclose their private medical information, and it's notable many of those who have 'come out' as disabled in recent years first did so through the necessity of cancelling a tour. And yet there is something undeniably moving about a musician being open about their disability if they choose to. It is not simply that celebrity culture means the act spreads awareness of a misunderstood condition (how many people learned about fibromyalgia by reading Lady Gaga had it?) but that it connects to others who are going through a similar experience. A teenage girl can be in bed crying from a pain spike and put on 'Poker Face' knowing her favourite artist understands. That means something.

Marina, formerly of Marina and the Diamonds, is one of the high-profile artists now speaking openly about their physical and mental health. In 2016, just as Marina was celebrating her third Top 10 album in the UK and first Top 10 entry on the US Billboard charts, behind the scenes she was starting to experience debilitating chronic fatigue. 'My energy levels dropped to around 50–60 per cent and I found myself choosing carefully between work and keeping some semblance of a social life. On tour, I would rest in the daytime and keep my schedule simple. I pushed myself too far many, many times until I started having severe flare-ups in 2023 that would take me ten days to recover from. I went through most of my flare-ups behind closed doors, isolating myself for as long as I needed to recover so team members weren't privy to how dysfunctional my life had become.'

Though Marina's health has thankfully improved recently, speaking out about her chronic illness on social media was a turning point for how she felt about it and the pressure to 'push through'. 'When I went public, the reaction was very supportive. I didn't expect that. I felt incredibly embarrassed to reveal the reality of my experience. Sharing my experience was an act of kindness and healing to myself. After keeping things hidden for so long, it felt like I had thrown open the windows and let the fresh air in. My feelings of embarrassment started to evaporate soon after that. I learned about the health struggles of fans I'd met who I never would have guessed were suffering with serious chronic conditions.

'If I think back to my first managers fifteen years ago, I don't think they were equipped to deal with conversations about mental or physical health. None of us were. Anything that meant I would have to pull out of something was a big no-no. The pressure for things to go well was huge. I went on tour with a vocal haemorrhage in 2012 because of this. It took a year of speech training to rehabilitate my voice again afterwards. I think there is a way to work and tour without pushing someone's wellbeing to the brink. It's not as complex as people imagine. Scheduling enough downtime between tours. Being mindful with the amount of travel and time-zone changes an artist is doing in a set period. Scheduling adequate time for recovery. I think so many artists are scared in the beginning to turn things down and instead compromise their health and personal life. "No" isn't a bad word.'

As this chapter has shown, there's still a stark lack of disability representation in the UK across anything from television, politics, fashion to music. I don't believe that fixing this will somehow solve the issues I've raised in this book. Representation is effectively 'trickle-down equality': focusing on it alone can obscure, rather than address, the day-to-day inequalities that shape disabled women's lives. Or to put it another way: wheelchair Barbie is not going to solve the pay gap.

And yet, as we have seen, there is still plenty to gain from having disabled women take our place at the forefront of mainstream culture. Representation pushes the edges of what is possible. Every disabled actor who has trail-blazed on to a screen in recent years, every politician who now speaks openly about their mental health, helps to normal-ize disability for non-disabled people while making those of us with a health condition feel that little bit more accepted. For all the shortcomings and frustrations, a disabled girl growing up today is able to switch on the TV and see someone who looks like her. That is not nothing.

Perhaps this progress will bound onwards to full equality. Or perhaps we will rest here for another fifty years, our backsides parked and boots dug firmly into the floor. I like to think we are moving forwards, even if the walk feels slow and tiring sometimes. Over recent decades, we – disabled women and our allies – have made strides in every aspect of society. We have gone from being hidden away in insti-tutions to shining on the front page of magazines, from the law of the land shutting us out of education and a career, to legislating ourselves in Parliament. The shift has been remarkable, really, and it will continue, bit by bit, step by step.

What it is to live with a disability or health condition cannot be boiled down to stereotypes or even shrunk to fit inside the pages of a book. It is a vast and varied experience, full of strength and anguish and private jokes that make your ribs hurt. But I hope these chapters have gone some way towards lifting such experiences into public view. Perhaps in the end, this book really is about representation – a project to collect the voices of women and non-binary people with disabilities and for the disabled community to, at least in a small way, see themselves reflected back. If the stories in *Who Wants Normal?* have shown one thing, it is that being seen matters. As women with physical or mental health conditions, there are few things more powerful than knowing the smallness and shame the world so often asks of us and refusing to apologize, shrink or change. Our lives should not be hidden. Our bodies do not belong behind closed doors. There is no such thing as normal. And if there was, we would have no obligation to conform to it. Disabled women, in all our uniqueness and glory, are pretty incredible as we are.

Final (wise) words

Rt Hon. Marsha de Cordova MP 'Follow your dreams and pursue your passions, even if you're afraid. Don't let your disability – or anyone's opinion – hold you back. Find yourself a good mentor and have a plan.'

Lara Parker 'Please, please don't waste any of your time thinking that you are wrong for being exactly the way you are. You are working in the only way you are able, and it is more than enough.'

Jillian Mercado 'You are not alone. There's going to be ups and downs and things in between that will hurt you and make you believe that there is no one going through the same things that you are. But I am here to tell you that we are here, that you are loved, and that we will stand behind you in any way possible. Being a woman who is disabled is an extra layer of being a woman. It definitely won't be easy, but I can assure you that you are resilient and you are so strong. You just have to know that you are and I can tell you for a fact that it will be all OK.'

Jenny Sealey OBE 'Find out about and get proper access. Hold your nerve. Don't be scared to get it wrong. Be curious always.'

Jameela Jamil 'You are smarter, more emotionally adept and stronger for what you have endured. You have empathy and perspective and therefore you have substance and a more interesting outlook. Just block out the nonsense, avoid magazines that avoid people like you and your experience. Avoid anyone who makes you feel lesser online. Fill your brain with what will nourish you rather than starve you of the self-respect you deserve. We are superior to those who do not have to endure the same things we do. Never forget this. You're fucking great and I'm extremely proud of you.'

Rosie Jones 'If you have a shot of whisky, and then you have a shot of pickle juice, it tastes *exactly* like a cheeseburger. Honestly, it does, try it. [That and . . .] be whoever you want to be. Having a disability is not a disadvantage; it's a different perspective. We all have our strengths and our weaknesses, and sometimes a weakness can become our biggest strength.'

Sinéad Burke 'You are a work in progress; your opinions, beliefs, thoughts, ambitions and the language you use to describe yourself and the world around you will evolve and change. We need to create space to not be continuously tied to what we once wanted, and to be open to an evolved perception of who we are, and what we want to become.'

Natasha Devon MBE 'Advocate for yourself and trust your instincts.'

Kelly Knox 'No matter what society or an individual may say, remember how unique, beautiful, valid and worthy you are to receive all the good this world has to offer. Don't let anyone strip you of your beauty, whatever your goals, dreams and ambitions are – you can achieve them. Being disabled is a gift! The way we do things on a daily basis makes us brilliant problem-solvers, adaptable, naturally creative and courageous. You've got to be pretty special to be in our club.'

Sarah Gordy MBE 'Life is about finding something you are interested in and enjoying it. It can be your job or something you do in your own time. Believe in yourself, take care of yourself and care for others. Smile a lot. Share happiness.'

Nadia Whittome MP 'I think there's a lot of shame and guilt that can come with having health conditions. If you've been let down by services or other institutions, know that that isn't your fault. How you feel or your inability to do certain things is also not your fault. You are dealing with a society that is not set up for your needs. You deserve to live a full and happy life, and the support to get there.'

Ruth Madeley 'You have no idea of the power you bring to the table. What you have to offer is unique and it's needed more than you know.'

Alice Wong 'Try not to feel the need to keep up or be as good as your non-disabled peers. Focus on doing what you love and knowing who you are and what kind of person you want to be in the world. Life can be messy and shitty and it's totally OK to be full of rage and pain. Don't do something because it's what others expect – please yourself first and take your time. You don't have to follow the typical path. You can find freedom when you let go of what you think success, perfection or happiness is supposed to look like. Asking for help and needing help doesn't mean you are a failure. You have power whether you realize it or not.'

Cherylee Houston MBE 'Do not take on-board what society thinks of you. As I've gotten older, I know that there's nothing wrong with being disabled. I now see it as a gift. I love being disabled and I believe it's given me a much richer life than one I would've had without it. The hardest thing about it is other people's opinions. But the more vocal you are the more they get over it.'

Dame Anne Begg 'Never doubt yourself. Making yourself heard as both a woman and with a disability will not be easy. Discrimination is sadly all too apparent. But everyone in society has a duty to both educate and help campaign for equality for all.'

Emma Barnett 'Learn a set routine of coping and take the energy when you have it to always ensure you have what you need to hand. Advocate for yourself, or find someone who can, to push doctors for diagnosis and then as much care as possible.'

Lucy Watts MBE 'You matter and you have great gifts to give to this world. Don't let anyone ever tell you that you cannot do something or let others' low expectations lower your own.'

Baroness Tanni Grey-Thompson 'Be proud of who you are. There will be people who will want to change you, people will have a view of what your life will be like. You have more choice in what you do than you realize.'

Josie George 'I want you to know that you can find a way to be happy and thrive in this body you're in. You don't have to try to be like anyone else: you can just be you. It will take time to figure out, but learning who you really are and how you want to express yourself can be really fun. Your story, your goals and your dreams might not play out how you think they will – and that's part of the adventure! – but just keep being your own best friend and know that your body is not your enemy. Be yourself all the way to your edges and good things will happen.'

Baroness Jane Campbell 'Never give up the fight for inclusion! Nothing will ever change about us, without us!'

Sophie Morgan 'Your disability can be your greatest opportunity to learn about the world, and although it's scary and tough at times, try and focus on what you can do instead of what you can't. The world around you will try and tell you that your life isn't worth as much as others' – don't believe them. Determine your own worth and live by your own beliefs. Ask for help when you need it.'

Fearne Cotton 'My advice might sound a little cheesy, but bear with me. I went to a Coldplay concert recently and on a big lit-up screen these words appeared. "If you want to be loved, be love". I stopped and stared at the screen. Isn't that what we all want? To be loved and seen? It's about trying to remember that we won't feel better if other people approve of us, or even love us, we have to feel that inside. That's where you can find peace. It doesn't mean you have to stand there shouting "I LOVE MYSELF" but it does mean if you can tap into that well of love that lives within you, then we in turn will be loved, and for all the right reasons. I wish I had known that growing up.'

Ione Gamble 'Do not fight your body, no matter how tempting it may be. Do not psychologically beat yourself up because you don't look the same, or can't do the same things as your peers. Find a rhythm that works for you in this world and try as hard as you can to be proud of it!'

Katie Piper OBE 'BE SEEN. I like that quote: "I am not what I've done or been through; I am what I've conquered and overcome." The fact is, pain builds resilience, patience and empathy in all of us. Worry is a total waste of time. It doesn't change anything. All it does is steal your joy and keep you very busy doing nothing.'

Stefanie Reid MBE 'You will always stand out with a disability. People may stare, people may think you are different to them, and people may be uncomfortable with you. And the best thing I've found is to own it! There is power in "otherness". I have experience and a perspective that no one else has and there is value in that. But only if I see it, and only if I believe it.'

Hannah Jane Parkinson 'I've noted of late that there's a sort of movement of people being "proud" of conditions. I think that is wonderful but I would also say that it's fine to be . . . well, pissed off. I would say it's OK to be low-key furious some of the time. But I would also say that there will be times when you feel much better – whether it's a mental or physical condition – and that things will be good. And during the bad times, there will be friends and family who are rooting for you. So, keep on keeping on, even when it's a total pain in the arse.'

Nikki Fox 'Do not ever limit yourself. The world isn't perfect by any stretch. A lot of things need to improve for disability, from the built environment to attitudes. But don't think too much about that shit. When I grew up, I was naive. I thought I could do anything. And actually, that helped me. Fake it until you make it. If I wanted a job, I didn't worry about how I'd do it; I just applied. At the same time, as I've got older, I've learned we have limits. Don't feel the pressure to be this unbelievable go-getter disabled person. That you have to try extra hard just because you're disabled. You don't have to. And it's not worth it.'

And from me . . . 'Your body does not need to shrink to fit the box of whatever "normal" is to have the right to enjoy any aspect of life. Thrive in your career while using adjustments that suit your needs. Have great sex in whatever way feels good to you. Put your favourite dress on for drinks with friends and then proudly pick up your cane. And know that millions of us are right there beside you cheering you on.'

Notes

Introduction

1. https://www.mirror.co.uk/news/uk-news/its-appalling-less-1-mps-27391412.amp
2. https://metro.co.uk/2018/09/12/as-a-disabled-comedian-i-know-how-much-things-could-change-if-there-were-people-like-me-on-tv-7937384/amp
3. https://bookriot.com/disability-representation-in-childrens-books/amp
4. https://www.thinkwithgoogle.com/intl/en-gb/future-of-marketing/management-and-culture/diversity-and-inclusion/how-rihannas-fenty-beauty-delivered-beauty-for-all-and-a-wake-up-call-to-the-industry/amp
5. https://amp.theguardian.com/commentisfree/2018/jan/07/vogue-new-suffragettes-women-disabilities
6. https://disabilityunit.blog.gov.uk/2021/07/28/shopping-national-disability-strategy-explained
7. https://www.ageukmobility.co.uk/mobility-news/article/how-accessible-is-the-uk
8. https://tfl.gov.uk/travel-information/improvements-and-projects/step-free-access
9. https://www.itv.com/news/2021-01-15/housing-crisis-for-disabled-people-set-to-deepen-report-finds

10. https://www.bbc.co.uk/news/uk-politics-30342957
11. https://amp.theguardian.com/society/2016/jul/19/people-with-disabilities-treated-like-second-class-citizens-says-watchdog
12. https://www.jrf.org.uk/report/uk-poverty-2019-20-social-security
13. https://www.tuc.org.uk/news/non-disabled-workers-paid-17-more-disabled-peers-tuc
14. https://www.independent.co.uk/news/uk/home-news/disabled-people-jobs-applications-more-able-bodied-stats-before-employment-a7970701.html
15. https://www.peoplemanagement.co.uk/article/1747045/most-business-leaders-apprehensive-hire-senior-disabled-employee
16. https://www.scope.org.uk/campaigns/extra-costs
17. https://amp.theguardian.com/society/2023/aug/17/ministers-failures-mean-disabled-people-in-uk-face-growing-poverty-risk-report
18. https://www.scope.org.uk/media/disability-facts-figures
19. https://www.scope.org.uk/scope/media/files/campaigns/disability-perception-gap-report.pdf
20. https://news.samsung.com/uk/new-research-reveals-nearly-half-of-the-nation-arent-comfortable-talking-about-disabilities-in-the-workplace
21. https://commonslibrary.parliament.uk/research-briefings/cbp-9602
22. https://commonslibrary.parliament.uk/research-briefings/cbp-9602
23. https://www.who.int/news-room/fact-sheets/detail/disability-and-health

24. https://www.scientificamerican.com/article/why-women-report-being-in

25. https://bmcwomenshealth.biomedcentral.com/articles/10.1186/s12905-021-01189-5#ref-CR1

26. https://amp.theguardian.com/uk-news/2023/feb/08/surge-in-young-people-declaring-disability-in-england-and-wales

27. https://amp.theguardian.com/society/2013/may/22/women-men-mental-illness-study

28. https://www.nature.com/articles/d41586-021-01836-9

29. https://www.hopkinsmedicine.org/health/conditions-and-diseases/multiple-sclerosis-ms/multiple-sclerosis-why-are-women-more-at-risk?amp=true

30. https://www.womenshealth.gov/a-z-topics/osteoporosis

School

1. https://assets.publishing.service.gov.uk/government/uploads/system/uploads/attachment_data/file/874507/family-resources-survey-2018-19.pdf

2. https://warwick.ac.uk/newsandevents/pressreleases/new_insights_into

3. https://www.ons.gov.uk/peoplepopulationandcommunity/healthandsocialcare/disability/articles/outcomesfordisabledpeopleintheuk/2020#education

4. There is little information available for how this breaks down for individual disabilities but what we do know shows a stark attainment gap. For example, research by the National Deaf Children's Society in 2021 showed that Deaf pupils in England achieve an entire GCSE grade less than their hearing

peers: https://www.ndcs.org.uk/about-us/news-and-media/latest-news/deaf-pupils-achieve-an-entire-gcse-grade-less-for-sixth-year-running

5. https://warwick.ac.uk/newsandevents/pressreleases/new_insights_into

6. education.https://amp.theguardian.com/education/article/2024/may/04/school-leaders-warn-of-full-blown-special-needs-crisis-in-england

7. https://www.theguardian.com/education/2019/may/07/cuts-heads-refuse-school-places-pupils-special-needs?CMP=Share_iOSApp_Other

8. https://www.independent.co.uk/news/education/education-news/teaching-assistants-funding-cuts-schools-headteachers-naht-austerity-a8248816.html

9. https://www.ndcs.org.uk/about-us/news-and-media/latest-news/yet-more-cuts-to-key-staff-as-deaf-children-fall-behind-at-school

10. https://www.mind.org.uk/news-campaigns/news/almost-two-thirds-of-young-people-receive-no-support-from-school-for-their-mental-health

11. https://inews.co.uk/news/education/parents-furious-government-drive-send-unwell-children-school-2896249

12. https://www.theguardian.com/education/2024/apr/15/parents-unwell-child-fear-truancy-prosecution

13. https://www.theguardian.com/education/2024/mar/29/aberdeen shire-pupils-with-complex-needs-erased-from-school-photo

14. https://warwick.ac.uk/newsandevents/pressreleases/new_insights_into

15. https://warwick.ac.uk/newsandevents/pressreleases/new_
    insights_into

16. https://journals.sagepub.com/doi/full/10.1177/0038038515574813

17. https://www.mind.org.uk/media/8852/not-making-the-grade.pdf

University

1. https://www.officeforstudents.org.uk/publications/beyond-
   the-bare-minimum-are-universities-and-colleges-doing-
   enough-for-disabled-students

2. https://www.ons.gov.uk/peoplepopulationandcommunity/
   healthandsocialcare/disability/articles/outcomesfordisabledpeo
   pleintheuk/2020#education

3. https://www.officeforstudents.org.uk/publications/beyond-
   the-bare-minimum-are-universities-and-colleges-doing-
   enough-for-disabled-students

4. https://www.officeforstudents.org.uk/media/1a263fd6-b20a-
   4ac7-b268-0bbaa0c153a2/beyond-the-bare-minimum-are-
   universities-and-colleges-doing-enough-for-disabled-students.
   pdf%252520/t%252520_blank

5. https://www.independent.co.uk/news/education/education-
   news/disabled-students-university-dropping-out-support-ofs-
   education-a9160416.html

6. https://www.officeforstudents.org.uk/publications/corona
   virus-briefing-note-disabled-students

7. https://www.tandfonline.com/doi/full/10.1080/09687599.2021
   .1907549

8. https://www.education-ni.gov.uk/articles/raise-programme

9. https://disabledstudents.co.uk

Careers

1. https://www.unison.org.uk/content/uploads/2013/07/On-line-Catalogue216953.pdf

2. https://www.unison.org.uk/motions/2021/conference-type/combating-bullying-and-harassment-of-disabled-workers-in-the-community-sector

3. https://www.tuc.org.uk/research-analysis/reports/sexual-harassment-disabled-women-workplace

4. https://www.tuc.org.uk/sites/default/files/SexualHarassmentreport2016.pdf

5. https://www.tuc.org.uk/research-analysis/reports/sexual-harassment-disabled-women-workplace

6. https://www.tes.com/magazine/archived/disabled-teachers-sidelined-and-told-get-it

7. https://www.bma.org.uk/media/2923/bma-disability-in-the-medical-profession.pdf

8. https://www.tortoisemedia.com/disability100-report

9. https://www.ft.com/content/e91c8785-8517-4f1a-b471-c80e80d6d8e2

10. https://www.ons.gov.uk/peoplepopulationandcommunity/healthandsocialcare/disability/bulletins/disabilityandemploymentuk/2019

11. time https://www.gov.uk/government/statistics/the-employment-of-disabled-people-2021/the-employment-of-disabled-people-2021

12. https://www.tuc.org.uk/research-analysis/reports/disability-pay-and-employment-gaps-2020

13. https://www.tuc.org.uk/news/tuc-3-4-disabled-workers-earn-less-ps15-hour

14. https://www.tuc.org.uk/research-analysis/reports/disability-pay-and-employment-gaps-2020

15. https://www.tuc.org.uk/news/tuc-slams-zero-progress-disability-pay-gap-last-decade

16. https://www.fenews.co.uk/employability/disability-inequity-at-work-22-of-business-leaders-unlikely-to-hire-candidates-with-known-disabilities

17. https://www.google.co.uk/amp/s/www.independent.co.uk/news/uk/home-news/disabled-people-jobs-applications-more-able-bodied-stats-before-employment-a7970701.html%3famp

18. https://amp.theguardian.com/careers/2015/may/06/how-to-use-your-disability-as-a-strength-when-applying-for-jobs

19. https://news.samsung.com/uk/new-research-reveals-nearly-half-of-the-nation-arent-comfortable-talking-about-disabilities-in-the-workplace

20. https://www.gov.uk/government/statistics/the-employment-of-disabled-people-2021/the-employment-of-disabled-people-2021

21. https://leonardcheshire.org/get-involved/campaign-us/employment

22. https://news.sky.com/story/one-in-three-may-struggle-to-make-ends-meet-in-retirement-report-warns-12910789

23. https://www.aeaweb.org/articles?id=10.1257/jel.20160995

24. https://amp.theguardian.com/world/2019/apr/04/gender-pay-gap-figures-show-eight-in-10-uk-firms-pay-men-more-than-women

25. https://www.tuc.org.uk/news/tuc-slams-zero-progress-disability-pay-gap-last-decade

26. https://www.tuc.org.uk/news/tuc-poll-two-five-disabled-workers-pushed-hardship-during-pandemic

27. https://www.tuc.org.uk/news/tuc-slams-zero-progress-disability-pay-gap-last-decade

28. https://www.scope.org.uk/campaigns/extra-costs

29. https://www.independent.co.uk/news/uk/home-news/pay-rise-women-work-awkward-gender-pay-gap-a9147931.html?amp

30. https://www.independent.co.uk/news/uk/home-news/pay-rise-women-work-awkward-gender-pay-gap-a9147931.html?amp

31. https://amp.theguardian.com/world/2022/apr/03/women-who-ask-for-pay-rise-less-successful-than-men-uk-poll-reveals

32. https://lweb.cfa.harvard.edu/cfawis/bowles.pdf

33. https://news.samsung.com/uk/new-research-reveals-nearly-half-of-the-nation-arent-comfortable-talking-about-disabilities-in-the-workplace

34. https://hrnews.co.uk/shhh-most-brits-prefer-not-to-talk-about-their-wages

35. https://www.peoplemanagement.co.uk/news/articles/two-five-disabled-workers-not-receiving-reasonable-adjustments-research-finds#gref

36. https://www.unison.org.uk/content/uploads/2021/10/Disabled-Members-annual-report-2020_21.pdf

37. https://www.ons.gov.uk/employmentandlabourmarket/peopleinwork/employmentandemployeetypes/articles/characteristicsofhomeworkersgreatbritain/september2022tojanuary2023

38. https://www.artsupplies.co.uk/blog/life-through-the-eyes-of-frida-kahlo

39. https://www.statista.com/statistics/1388245/uk-sick-leave-figures

40. https://amp.theguardian.com/society/2023/dec/24/500000-under-35s-out-of-work-long-term-illness-uk

41. https://www.health.org.uk/news-and-comment/news/300000-people-leave-the-workforce-and-report-ill-health-annually

42. https://news.sky.com/story/amp/number-of-long-term-sick-hits-record-high-of-2-6-million-12959783

43. https://www.thetimes.com/uk/politics/article/young-women-more-likely-to-be-out-of-work-sick-than-with-children-nq7x2h2d8

44. https://metro.co.uk/2022/03/21/benefits-street-star-white-dee-accuses-channel-4-of-exploiting-cast-16313141/amp

45. https://www.indy100.com/amp/the-daily-mail-has-admitted-its-story-about-disability-scheme-fraud-was-wrong-7299276-2656359585

46. https://amp.theguardian.com/politics/2013/jan/08/strivers-shirkers-language-welfare

47. https://amp.theguardian.com/uk-news/2023/nov/21/disabled-people-work-from-home-laura-trott-benefits

48. https://www.scope.org.uk/media/disability-facts-figures

49. https://hbr.org/2015/04/why-some-men-pretend-to-work-80-hour-weeks

50. https://www.nber.org/papers/w22365

51. https://hbr.org/2015/04/working-long-hours-makes-us-drink-more

52. https://autonomy.work/wp-content/uploads/2020/10/4DW-mentalhealth_cumpass_4dwcORANGE_C-v2.pdf

53. https://www.linkedin.com/news/story/burnout-at-work-is-on-the-rise-6173210

54. https://www.forbes.com/sites/markcperna/2023/12/12/meet-the-latest-version-of-quiet-quitting-lazy-girl-jobs

Body Image

1. https://www.chronicmom.com/2021/08/how-the-ugly-laws-were-designed-to-keep-disabled-people-out-of-sight.html

2. https://www.telegraph.co.uk/news/uknews/1458481/Anger-over-freak-show-pictures-of-midgets-the-deformed-and-the-fat.html

3. https://www.bbc.com/news/newsbeat-49662140.amp

4. https://www.leonardcheshire.org/about-us/our-news/press-releases/disability-hate-crimes-rise-record-levels

5. https://www.bbc.co.uk/news/newsbeat-61464341

6. https://graziadaily.co.uk/beauty-hair/wellness/disabled-women-groping-harassment

7. https://committees.parliament.uk/publications/2691/documents/26657/default

8. https://www.tandfonline.com/doi/abs/10.1080/00380237.2003.10570722

9. https://www.koimoi.com/hollywood-news/selena-gomez-shells-out-queen-behaviour-giving-a-savage-response-to-tiktok-user-defending-her-weight-gain-in-viral-bikini-videos-i-love-my-body-watch/amp

10. https://pubmed.ncbi.nlm.nih.gov/30793457

11. https://amp.theguardian.com/film/2022/apr/20/liza-minnelli-was-sabotaged-at-oscars-and-forced-to-appear-in-wheelchair

12. https://disabilityunit.blog.gov.uk/2021/07/28/shopping-national-disability-strategy-explained

13. https://disabilityunit.blog.gov.uk/2021/07/28/shopping-national-disability-strategy-explained

14. https://www.bbc.co.uk/news/uk-politics-30342957.amp

15. https://www.retailgazette.co.uk/blog/2024/01/primark-adaptive-fashion

16. https://youtu.be/B_P9pu8gytl

17. https://www.drapersonline.com/news/primark-unveils-adaptive-clothing-line-with-victoria-jenkins? utm_source=WordPress&utm_medium=Recommendation&utm_campaign=Recommended_Articles

18. https://www.theguardian.com/business/article/2024/aug/10/m-and-s-sells-knickers-designed-to-be-worn-with-stoma-in-uk-high-street-first

19. https://unhiddenclothing.com

20. https://www.retailgazette.co.uk/blog/2024/01/primark-adaptive-fashion

21. https://wearepurple.org.uk/the-purple-pound-infographic

22. https://wearepurple.org.uk/the-purple-pound-infographic

23. https://pubmed.ncbi.nlm.nih.gov/7636772

24. https://www.researchgate.net/publication/271666578_Body_Image_among_Women_with_Physical_Disabilities_Internalization_of_Norms_and_Reactions_to_Nonconformity

Healthcare

1. https://www.healthaffairs.org/doi/10.1377/hlthaff.2022.00475

2. Galli, G., Lenggenhager, B., Scivoletto, G., et al., '"Don't look at my wheelchair!" The plasticity of longlasting prejudice', *Medical Education* (2015), 49: 1239–47.

3. https://www.healthaffairs.org/doi/10.1377/hlthaff.2020.01452

4. https://www.urban.org/research/publication/four-ten-adults-disabilities-experienced-unfair-treatment-health-care-settings

5. https://www.mencap.org.uk/learning-disability-explained/research-and-statistics/health/health-inequalities

6. https://www.mencap.org.uk/learning-disability-explained/research-and-statistics/health/health-inequalities

7. https://www.theguardian.com/society/2020/apr/01/ventilators-may-be-taken-from-stable-coronavirus-patients-for-healthier-ones-bma-says?CMP=Share_iOSApp_Other

8. https://www.independent.co.uk/news/health/coronavirus-nhs-treatment-disabled-autism-nice-covid-19-a9423441.html

9. https://amp.theguardian.com/world/2021/feb/13/new-do-not-resuscitate-orders-imposed-on-covid-19-patients-with-learning-difficulties

10. https://www.bbc.co.uk/news/health-56435428.amp

11. https://globalgenes.org/2013/04/10/rare-disease-impact-report-quantifies-patient-and-caregiver-challenges

12. https://www.webmd.com/multiple-sclerosis/news/20210625/first-signs-of-ms-may-often-go-undiagnosed

13. https://amp.theguardian.com/society/2012/jun/27/bipolar-disorder-diagnosis-survey

14. https://www.healthdata.org/news-events/newsroom/news-releases/lancet-public-health-global-study-reveals-stark-differences

15. https://www.scientificamerican.com/article/why-women-report-being-in

16. https://www.reuters.com/article/us-health-diagnoses-gender-idUSKCN1R62IJ

17. https://www.bbc.com/future/article/20180523-how-gender-bias-affects-your-healthcare

18. https://www.verywellhealth.com/autism-diagnosis-adulthood-mental-health-5205054

19. https://www.bbc.com/future/article/20180523-how-gender-bias-affects-your-healthcare

20. Women even face a delay in being diagnosed for life-threatening conditions. A 2015 study (https://journals.plos.org/plosone/article?id=10.1371/journal.pone.0127717) revealed a longer time from the onset of symptoms to diagnosis in female patients in six out of eleven types of cancer. Notably the research showed it isn't that women wait longer to seek medical attention – the delay in diagnosis occurs after they've first visited their GP.

21. https://www.gov.uk/government/consultations/womens-health-strategy-call-for-evidence/outcome/results-of-the-womens-health-lets-talk-about-it-survey

22. As Evans says, it is not a coincidence that conditions that are more prevalent in women are the ones that are less likely to be taken seriously by medics. Autoimmune diseases like lupus, of which 90 per cent of patients are women (https://www.lupus.org/resources/lupus-facts-and-statistics), chronic pain conditions like fibromyalgia, of which 80–90 per cent of diagnosed cases are women (https://www.iasp-pain.org/advocacy/global-year/pain-in-women), and energy-related illnesses like ME, which affects women at a ratio of four to one (https://www.meresearch.org.uk/sex-differences-in-mecfs), are notoriously classified by medics as undetermined, psychological (https://meassociation.

org.uk/2016/06/the-all-in-the-mind-myth-of-myalgic-encephalomyelitis-chronic-fatigue-syndrome-nursing-in-practice-27-june-2016), or even 'fake'.

23. Another survey of more than 2,400 US women with a variety of chronic pain conditions found 91 per cent felt that the healthcare system discriminates against female patients. Nearly half were told the pain they experienced was all in their head: https://www.washingtonpost.com/health/is-bias-keeping-female-minority-patients-from-getting-proper-care-for-their-pain/2019/07/26/9d1b3a78-a810-11e9-9214-246e594de5d5_story.html

24. https://bmjopen.bmj.com/content/7/8/e016614

25. https://chronicillnessinclusion.org.uk/wp-content/uploads/2021/06/CII.DHSC-Womens-Health-England-June-2021.pdf

26. https://www.sense.org.uk/information-and-advice/for-professionals/policy-public-affairs-and-research/potential-and-possibility-research/access-to-healthcare

27. https://journals.sagepub.com/doi/full/10.1177/26330040211022033

28. https://www.neural.org.uk/wp-content/uploads/2022/05/Together-for-the-1-in-6-UK-Findings-from-My-Neuro-Survey-v6.pdf

29. https://www.kingsfund.org.uk/insight-and-analysis/blogs/nhs-spending-squeezed

30. https://www.bma.org.uk/advice-and-support/nhs-delivery-and-workforce/pressures/nhs-backlog-data-analysis

31. https://www.theguardian.com/society/2023/jul/24/most-nhs-staff-say-they-dont-have-enough-time-to-spend-with-patients

32. https://nhsproviders.org/news-blogs/blogs/the-issue-nobody-is-talking-about-that-could-decide-the-next-election

33. https://www.mind.org.uk/news-campaigns/news/mind-responds-to-uk-government-nhs-elective-recovery-plan

34. https://www.stonewall.org.uk/about-us/media-releases/stonewall-report-reveals-impact-discrimination-health-lgbt-people

35. https://dredf.org/health-disparities-at-the-intersection-of-disability-and-gender-identity/#_ednref34

36. https://www.independent.co.uk/news/uk/home-news/black-britons-discrimination-doctors-nurses-b2173959.html

37. https://academic.oup.com/painmedicine/article/13/2/150/1935962

38. https://pubmed.ncbi.nlm.nih.gov/27044069

39. https://www.theguardian.com/society/2022/aug/10/obese-patients-weight-shamed-doctors-nurses

40. https://www.ncbi.nlm.nih.gov/pmc/articles/PMC5386399

41. https://chronicillnessinclusion.org.uk

42. https://winvisible.org

43. https://butudontlooksick.com/about-me

44. https://www.who.int/publications/i/item/9789240063600

45. https://themighty.com/topic/disability/how-ableism-affects-mental-health-disability

46. https://www.disabilityrightsuk.org/news/2020/february/nearly-half-everyone-poverty-either-disabled-person-or-lives-disabled-person

47. https://www.leonardcheshire.org/about-us/our-news/press-releases/disabled-people-doubt-equality-act-decade

48. https://www.engender.org.uk/news/blog/disabled-womens-reproductive-rights-routinely-ignored

49. https://www.jostrust.org.uk/our-research-and-policy-work/our-research/barriers-cervical-screening-physical-disabilities

50. *Health and care of people with learning disabilities, experimental statistics* (2020), NHS Digital.

51. https://www.nhs.uk/conditions/breast-screening-mammogram/when-youll-be-invited-and-who-should-go

52. https://news.cancerresearchuk.org/2017/09/29/women-with-disabilities-may-be-missing-out-on-cancer-screening

Relationships

1. https://www.intechopen.com/chapters/82075

2. https://www.tandfonline.com/doi/full/10.3109/09638280903419277

3. https://blog.scope.org.uk/2016/02/11/scopes-romance-classics

4. Scope with Opinium Polling Ltd (2022); unreleased research.

5. https://www.reuters.com/article/idUSTRE5AB0C5

6. https://www.bbc.com/news/newsbeat-62812834.amp

7. Notably, Ghouri later said her appearance on the programme led to online trolling in which viewers mocked her voice to the extent it trended on social media. https://www.bbc.com/news/articles/coj8zevz4gno.amp

8. https://disabilityhorizons.com/2021/06/itvs-announcement-of-first-disabled-contestant-on-love-island-sparks-mixed-opinions

9. https://www.mirror.co.uk/tv/tv-news/undateables-branded-offensive-exploitative-doctors-5940488.amp

10. https://www.teenvogue.com/story/the-metoo-movement-hasnt-been-inclusive-of-the-disability-community

11. https://amp.theguardian.com/commentisfree/2018/mar/08/disabled-people-metoo-womens-movement-inclusion-diversity

12. https://www.bbc.co.uk/news/articles/cvgdze14xzno.amp

13. https://www.womensaid.org.uk/information-support/the-survivors-handbook/the-survivors-handbook-disabled-women

14. https://www.bbc.co.uk/news/uk-46371441.amp

15. https://www.dailyrecord.co.uk/lifestyle/money/new-calls-dwp-benefit-rules-30249747.amp

16. https://www.theguardian.com/lifeandstyle/2016/feb/21/disabled-dating-tinder-sex-wheelchair-romance?CMP=Share_iOSApp_Other

17. https://uk.tinderpressroom.com/WELCOME-TO-A-RENAISSANCE-IN-DATING,-DRIVEN-BY-AUTHENTICITY

18. https://amp.theguardian.com/lifeandstyle/2014/apr/20/lets-talk-about-sex-education-disability

19. https://splitbanana.co.uk

20. https://www.elitedaily.com/dating/sex/faking-orgasms-partner-dump-you/1825534

21. lxxxhttps://twitter.com/jenlrossman/status/989258951517753344?s=46&t=MEwb9I1lPirXEJ79uW2WQA

22. https://www.dailyecho.co.uk/news/9774744.amp

23. https://www.bbc.co.uk/news/uk-39575293.amp

24. https://www.morningadvertiser.co.uk/Article/2023/03/29/how-accessible-are-pubs-and-bars-for-disabled-people

25. https://www.thespiritsbusiness.com/2019/03/survey-pubs-and-bars-harder-to-access-than-castles

26. https://www.leonardcheshire.org/our-impact/stories/why-are-there-so-few-accessible-lgbtq-venues

27. https://www.disabilityrightsuk.org/news/poll-reveals-extent-Loneliness-disabled-people

28. https://www.scope.org.uk/campaigns/research-policy/attitudes-towards-disabled-people

29. https://amp.theguardian.com/commentisfree/2023/may/29/you-dont-have-to-be-alone-to-experience-loneliness-and-more-friends-isnt-the-answer

30. https://www.disabilityrightsuk.org/news/poll-reveals-extent-Loneliness-disabled-people

31. https://www.disabilityrightsuk.org/news/poll-reveals-extent-Loneliness-disabled-people

32. http://enablemagazine.co.uk/nearly-half-disabled-people-feel-chronically-lonely

33. https://www.bbc.co.uk/news/blogs-ouch-31421248

34. https://www.scope.org.uk/media/press-releases/brits-feel-uncomfortable-with-disabled-people

35. https://www.sense.org.uk/media/latest-press-releases/loneliness-rises-dramatically-among-disabled-people

36. https://www.scope.org.uk/media/press-releases/scope-reveals-shocking-levels-of-online-trolling-experienced-by-disabled-people

Representation

1. https://committees.parliament.uk/publications/2691/documents/26657/default

2. https://creativediversitynetwork.com/wp-content/uploads/2022/03/TheFifthCut-Diamond-at-5.pdf

3. https://www.screenskills.com/media/5074/2nd-december-underlying-health-condition-report-tv.pdf

4. https://radiotoday.co.uk/2021/11/more-women-and-people-with-disabilities-are-leaving-radio-than-joining

5. https://www.channel4.com/press/news/channel-4-challenges-uk-advertisers-improve-disabled-representation-advertising-1

6. https://www.televisual.com/news/report-disabled-people-wont-be-properly-represented-in-tv-until-2041

7. https://www.televisual.com/news/report-disabled-people-wont-be-properly-represented-in-tv-until-2041

8. https://www.mirror.co.uk/3am/celebrity-news/cherylee-houston-makes-history-as-coronation-223123

9. https://amp.theguardian.com/society/2011/feb/21/tv-presenter-cerrie-burnell

10. https://news.sky.com/story/amp/disabled-workers-in-uk-television-industry-facing-barriers-to-career-progression-new-report-says-12388632

11. https://www.screenskills.com/media/5074/2nd-december-underlying-health-condition-report-tv.pdf

12. https://amp.theguardian.com/tv-and-radio/2023/apr/25/how-melanie-sykes-quit-tv-after-bad-treatment-by-men

13. https://the-media-leader.com/ofcom-more-women-are-leaving-tv-and-radio-than-joining

14. https://www.latimes.com/entertainment-arts/movies/story/2023-08-17/usc-annenberg-study-2007-2022-movies-hollywood-diversity

15. https://rudermanfoundation.org/white_papers/employment-of-actors-with-disabilities-in-television

16. https://www.indiewire.com/2017/09/actors-oscar-nominations-disabilities-afflictions

17. https://movieweb.com/inspiring-stories-disabled-actors-oscars

18. https://www.ted.com/talks/stella_young_i_m_not_your_inspiration_thank_you_very_much

19. https://www.screenskills.com/media/5074/2nd-december-underlying-health-condition-report-tv.pdf

20. https://commonslibrary.parliament.uk/research-briefings/sn06652

21. https://www.mirror.co.uk/news/uk-news/its-appalling-less-1-mps-27391412.amp

22. https://amp.theguardian.com/politics/2016/jul/26/kirsty-blackman-snp-mp-westminster-parliament-childcare-london

23. https://www.gov.uk/government/publications/ barriers_to_elected_office_for_disabled-people

24. https://amp.theguardian.com/politics/2023/sep/18/dehenna-davison-resigns-as-uk-minister-citing-struggle-with-chronic-migraine

25. https://www.forbes.com/sites/saradorn/2023/09/26/biden-slips-on-air-force-one-stairs-as-his-team-tries-to-prevent-major-falls-as-trips-and-gaffes-raise-concerns-about-his-age

26. https://www.bostonglobe.com/2024/03/12/opinion/joe-biden-age-slow-walk

27. https://www.telegraph.co.uk/royal-family/2023/04/08/queen-elizabeth-platinum-jubilee-wheelchair-robert-jobson

28. https://www.nps.gov/articles/disabilityhistorypresidents

29. https://www.thenational.scot/news/23316235.bbc-presenter-james-naughtie-claims-nicola-sturgeon-looking-tired

30. https://www.amnesty.org.uk/online-violence-women-mps

31. https://www.theguardian.com/politics/2023/nov/14/therese-coffey-says-she-nearly-died-from-ministerial-stress

32. https://www.gov.uk/government/publications/ barriers_to_elected_office_for_disabled-people

33. https://www.independent.co.uk/news/uk/politics/disability-shut-out-parliament-tories-access-elected-office-fund-labour-a8380576.html

34. https://www.theguardian.com/world/2022/jul/31/spain-beach-bodies-ad-edited-out-my-prosthetic-leg-says-british-model

35. https://www.theguardian.com/world/2022/jul/31/spain-beach-bodies-ad-edited-out-my-prosthetic-leg-says-british-model

36. https://www.dazeddigital.com/fashion/article/60230/1/disabled-representation-on-the-runway-fashion-campaign-catwalk-curve-poc-trans

37. https://www.british-fashioncouncil.co.uk/uploads/files/1/The us fashion DEI Report – 22.01.24.pdf

38. https://www.glamourmagazine.co.uk/article/shelby-lynch-self-love-january-2023

39. https://www.itv.com/news/2023-04-24/british-vogues-disabled-cover-stars-hope-to-spark-real-change-with-latest-issue

40. https://amp.theguardian.com/music/2023/jun/24/lewis-capaldi-at-glastonbury-review

41. https://fortune.com/well/2023/03/03/justin-bieber-ramsay-hunt-syndrome

42. https://www.musicweek.com/media/read/new-survey-by-attitude-is-everything-reveals-the-hidden-barriers-faced-by-disabled-musicians-and-artists

43. https://attitudeiseverything.org.uk/attitude-is-everything-and-black-lives-in-music-release-unseen-unheard-report-and-podcast

44. https://www.express.co.uk/celebrity-news/1854826/sam-smith-leg-brace-walking-stick-break-up-Christian-Cowan/amp

45. https://www.express.co.uk/celebrity-news/1519329/Elton-John-walking-stick-honour-Prince-Charles-surgery-health-Order-of-the-Companions-news/amp

46. https://www.ndtv.com/entertainment/jessie-j-almost-lost-ability-to-walk-after-breaking-her-ankle-613705/amp

47. https://www.billboard.com/music/music-news/chris-martin-pianist-one-hand-duet-video-1235128451/amp

48. https://www.drakemusic.org/about-us

49. https://www.bbc.co.uk/news/entertainment-arts-50247373.amp

50. https://oldtimemusic.com/the-meaning-behind-the-song-black-dog-by-arlo-parks

51. https://www.today.com/today/amp/rcna98154

52. https://www.harpersbazaar.com/celebrity/latest/a30414700/lady-gaga-oprah-interview-psychotic-break-chronic-illness

Index